Liquid Biopsy for Cancer

Seung Il Kim • Young Kim

Liquid Biopsy for Cancer

Current Status and Future Challenges

Springer

Seung Il Kim
Department of Surgery
Yonsei University College of Medicine
Seoul, Korea (Republic of)

Young Kim
Department of Surgery
Yonsei University College of Medicine
Seoul, Korea (Republic of)

ISBN 978-981-99-4417-0   ISBN 978-981-99-4418-7 (eBook)
https://doi.org/10.1007/978-981-99-4418-7

The original submitted manuscript has been translated into English. The translation was done using artificial intelligence. A subsequent revision was performed by the author(s) to further refine the work and to ensure that the translation is appropriate concerning content and scientific correctness. It may, however, read stylistically different from a conventional translation.

This Springer imprint is published by the registered company Springer Nature Singapore Pte Ltd.
The registered company address is: 152 Beach Road, #21-01/04 Gateway East, Singapore 189721, Singapore

Preface

Over the past two decades, the concept of liquid biopsy has evolved from an exploratory research topic into one of the most transformative paradigms in modern oncology. Once regarded merely as a complementary diagnostic approach, it now represents a cornerstone of precision medicine—enabling real-time, noninvasive access to the molecular landscape of tumors through a simple blood draw. Yet, despite its rapid conceptual rise, the path to full clinical realization has been far from linear. The translation of liquid biopsy from bench to bedside has demanded not only technological innovation but also rigorous analytical and clinical validation and interpretive precision rooted in biological understanding.

This book, *Liquid Biopsy for Cancer: Current Status and Future Challenges*, was conceived to provide an integrated and comprehensive view of this rapidly advancing field. It is the culmination of nearly two decades of clinical experience in breast cancer surgery and more than a decade of translational research focused on circulating biomarkers—specifically circulating tumor cells (CTCs), circulating tumor DNA (ctDNA), and extracellular vesicles (EVs). Through this synthesis, the book seeks to bridge the gap between the theoretical promise of liquid biopsy and its tangible clinical utility. The motivation for writing this book stems from a fundamental question that persists in every oncology clinic: *How can we understand and respond to the molecular evolution of cancer without performing repeated invasive biopsies?* Cancer is not a static disease but a dynamic and adaptive process. Each patient's tumor evolves continuously—responding to treatment, resisting stress, and reshaping its biology to survive. Traditional tissue biopsies, while critical for initial diagnosis, provide only a single temporal and spatial snapshot of the disease. Liquid biopsy, in contrast, allows for serial and systemic monitoring that reflects tumor heterogeneity and evolution in real time. It transforms how we observe, interpret, and ultimately intervene in the course of cancer progression. Realizing this vision, however, has required overcoming significant challenges. Each analyte—CTCs, ctDNA, and EVs—carries its own biological meaning, stability profile, and methodological complexity. CTCs provide a cellular mirror of metastatic potential; ctDNA offers real-time insight into genomic and epigenetic alterations; and EVs represent a rich and complex compartment that encapsulates the biochemical language of tumor–host communication. Only by integrating these multiple analytes can we begin to construct a truly multidimensional understanding of cancer biology and its clinical manifestations. Among these, extracellular vesicles (EVs), an area of our active investigation, have recently emerged as one of the most dynamic and promising analytes. Once dismissed as inert cellular debris, they are now recognized as key mediators of intercellular communication and as potent vehicles for diagnostic and therapeutic applications. EVs embody the dual nature of liquid biopsy—offering information for disease detection while simultaneously opening avenues for therapeutic delivery and molecular targeting. Their evolution from scientific skepticism to clinical relevance epitomizes the broader maturation of the field itself.

This book is not intended merely as a compilation of existing literature. It aims to serve as a bridge between molecular discovery, clinical implementation, and regulatory science, integrating perspectives from biology, oncology, bioengineering, and data science. It was written for a diverse readership: clinicians striving to incorporate liquid biopsy into precision oncology, laboratory scientists developing next-generation assays, graduate students entering this field, and industry or regulatory professionals seeking translational insight. Above all, it is intended for readers who share the conviction that the management of cancer must evolve toward real-time, patient-specific, and data-informed decision-making. Throughout this book, readers will find not only detailed scientific discussion but also reflections on the practical realities of translational medicine. The content reflects both the achievements and the challenges we have faced: moments when promising biomarkers failed validation, when reproducibility faltered, and when regulatory structures struggled to keep pace with innovation. These experiences have underscored a central principle that guides this work—progress in liquid biopsy depends not only on technological capability but on biological insight, methodological rigor, and multidisciplinary collaboration. The writing of this book also reflects the evolving nature of cancer research itself, which is no longer confined within traditional disciplinary boundaries. Today, the development of diagnostic and therapeutic technologies requires the combined expertise of clinicians, molecular biologists, engineers, and data scientists. The convergence of these disciplines allows us to move beyond static classification and toward dynamic modeling of disease behavior. The field of liquid biopsy, in particular, stands at this intersection—where biology meets technology, and where innovation must meet regulation. The completion of this book coincides with an era of unprecedented momentum. Multi-cancer early detection (MCED) platforms are being tested in large-scale clinical trials; minimal residual disease (MRD) detection is reshaping adjuvant therapy and surveillance strategies; and liquid biopsy–based companion diagnostics are receiving regulatory approvals across the globe. Yet these rapid advances also highlight a pressing need for harmonized standards, data-sharing frameworks, and interpretive guidelines to ensure that laboratory findings translate into meaningful patient outcomes. Our hope is that this volume will serve as both a scientific compass and a practical guide, helping readers navigate the opportunities and limitations inherent in this transformative field.

The journey of producing this book has also been deeply personal. It represents years of collective effort and collaboration among clinicians, basic scientists, engineers, and regulatory experts—individuals united by a shared vision of turning molecular insight into clinical benefit. It also reflects the dedication of a new generation of physician-scientists who transcend disciplinary boundaries and bridge the gap between discovery and application. Their curiosity, creativity, and perseverance have been the driving force behind every chapter. As we look toward the future, it is evident that oncology will no longer be defined by static tumor classifications or single-timepoint measurements. The next era will be characterized by dynamic, integrative, and patient-centered oncology, where continuous molecular profiling informs therapeutic decisions and predictive modeling replaces reactive treatment. Liquid biopsy—spanning from early diagnosis to therapeutic monitoring—will undoubtedly play a central role in this transformation. It is our hope that the knowledge compiled in this book will inspire further inquiry, foster interdisciplinary collaboration, and contribute to the realization of precision medicine as a tangible clinical reality.

Seoul, South Korea Seung Il Kim
Seoul, South Korea Young Kim

Contents

Liquid Biopsy in the Era of Precision Oncology

1

1.1 Tumor Heterogeneity as a Barrier to Therapeutic Success

The most fundamental cause of cancer treatment failure lies in the fact that tumors are not homogeneous entities, but rather complex and dynamic ecosystems that continuously evolve and differentiate. Tumors are biological conglomerates composed of various subclones—cellular subpopulations with distinct genetic and phenotypic characteristics—a phenomenon known as tumor heterogeneity. This heterogeneity can be broadly categorized along two axes: spatial and temporal (Fig. 1.1).

Intratumoral spatial heterogeneity refers to the phenomenon in which cells located in different regions of the same tumor harbor distinct genetic mutations or exhibit variable responses to therapy. In other words, even within a single tumor, cells at the core, the periphery, perivascular regions, and hypoxic zones may each possess unique genetic alterations or metabolic profiles. For example, cells at the tumor core may adapt to hypoxic conditions by overexpressing HIF (hypoxia-inducible factor) signaling, while those at the periphery may represent highly invasive clones.

These differences ultimately result in variable drug responsiveness depending on tumor location.

Temporal heterogeneity refers to the phenomenon in which tumors continuously evolve (dynamic tumor evolution) and acquire resistance mutations under external pressures such as anticancer therapy. Initially, drug-sensitive clones may disappear over time, while a small population of resistant clones can emerge as the dominant group, leading to recurrence. Such heterogeneity enables cancer to acquire resistance to anticancer agents and forms the biological basis for recurrence and metastasis. These changes demonstrate that cancer is not a single disease entity, but rather a condition that continuously evolves throughout the course of treatment.

Furthermore, tumor heterogeneity extends beyond simple genetic diversity and is closely linked to the influence of the tumor microenvironment (TME). The TME comprises immune cells, fibroblasts, and vascular endothelial cells, which interact to accelerate tumor evolution. Differences between patients who respond to immune checkpoint inhibitors and those who do not are ultimately the result of the complex interplay between the TME and tumor heterogeneity. In this respect, understanding tumor heterogeneity is not limited to the tumor itself, but involves comprehending the triangular relationship among the tumor, microenvironment, and therapeutics.

Recent advances in single-cell genomics and spatial transcriptomics have enabled the quantification and visualization of tumor heterogeneity. These technologies have demonstrated that, even within tumors from the same patient, distinct subclones may follow different evolutionary tra-

S. I. Kim, Y. Kim, *Liquid Biopsy for Cancer*, https://doi.org/10.1007/978-981-99-4418-7_1

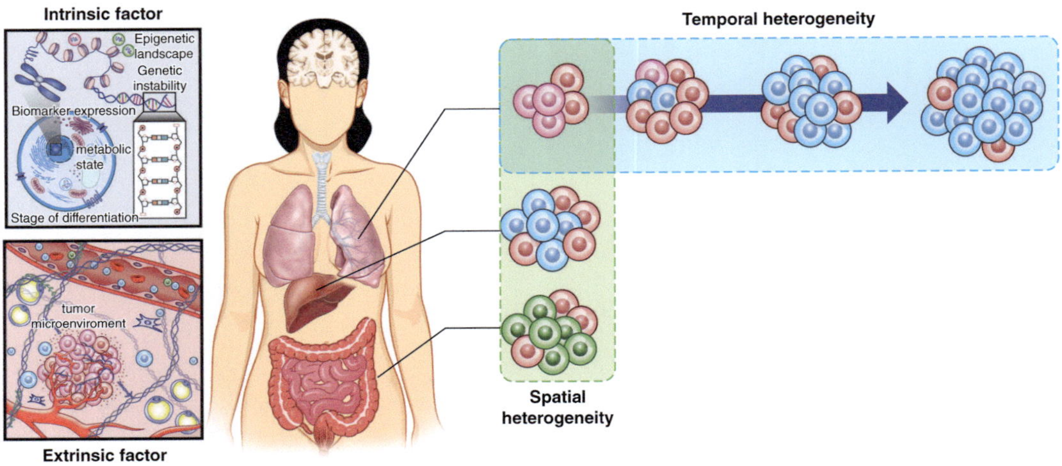

Fig. 1.1 Tumor heterogeneity characterized by the temporal and spatial distribution of tumors, regulated by intrinsic and extrinsic factors

jectories, resulting in variable therapeutic responses. Notably, the clonal evolution model proposed by McGranahan and Swanton describes tumors as continuously evolving ecosystems, highlighting the importance of considering spatiotemporal context when selecting therapeutic targets in precision medicine.

To improve outcomes in cancer therapy, it is insufficient to rely solely on strategies based on a single time point or a single sample. Cancer is not a static entity, but a dynamic network. It continuously evolves through interactions among the tumor, the microenvironment, and the immune system. As a result, cancer precision medicine must evolve into a dynamic treatment decision system that integratively analyzes the spatiotemporal heterogeneity of tumors. This is the fundamental rationale for the growing need for liquid biopsy. It represents a core theme in cancer precision medicine in the modern genome-driven oncology era.

1.2 Limitations of Tissue Biopsy: Can It Capture Spatial and Temporal Heterogeneity?

Tissue biopsy has long been the standard for cancer diagnosis and molecular analysis. However, considering tumor heterogeneity, tissue biopsy has inherent limitations. It is well known that tissue biopsy, which involves sampling a small portion of tissue from a specific site, cannot fully reflect the overall heterogeneity of the tumor. In particular, tissue obtained by core needle biopsy represents only a specific region of the tumor and is unlikely to capture the full clonal diversity. Even surgical specimens provide information only at a specific "pre-treatment" time point and do not reflect evolutionary and resistance changes that occur during therapy. The situation is even more complex in metastatic cancer. In metastatic disease, lesions in different organs may harbor distinct molecular characteristics, and capturing this diversity would require invasive and repeated tissue biopsies, which are neither clinically feasible nor acceptable to patients.

These limitations are clearly evident in clinical practice. For example, when repeated tissue biopsies are performed on deep lung lesions in lung cancer patients, the risk of complications such as pneumothorax, hemorrhage, and infection has been reported to be as high as 20–30% [1]. In addition, patients may refuse the procedure due to fear and discomfort. Ultimately, the greatest limitation of tissue biopsy is that it provides only a static snapshot. Cancer evolves continuously over months and years, whereas tissue biopsy provides information only from a fixed location at a single point in time. In contrast, patients experience dynamic processes such as treatment, recurrence, and the development of resistance. Consequently, clinicians are faced with the paradox of having to manage a constantly changing disease based on historical information. Due to these limitations, staging and treatment decisions for patients often rely on limited sample information, which reduces the accuracy of predicting therapeutic response. Therefore, to capture tumor heterogeneity and track dynamic tumor evolution in real time, a more continuous and noninvasive alternative is needed—this is the context in which liquid biopsy emerged.

1.3 Emergence of Liquid Biopsy: A Paradigm Shift in Oncology

Consider a lung cancer patient who must undergo a high-risk procedure to access a deep region of the lung for tissue biopsy. Repeat procedures are not feasible, and assessment of treatment response must rely on fragmentary information from the initial tissue sample. What if treatment response could be monitored and recurrence detected early with a simple blood test? What if treatment strategies could be adjusted in a timely manner while minimizing patient burden? The technology that makes this possible is liquid biopsy, and today its potential is no longer theoretical but a clinical reality. As an alternative to overcome the limitations of traditional tissue-based diagnostic methods, liquid biopsy using circulating cancer biomarkers in blood has recently gained attention. The concept of liquid biopsy originated from the idea that circulating cancer biomarkers, released into the bloodstream from tumors composed of various clones, could integratively reflect the molecular biological information of the tumor and represent its spatiotemporal heterogeneity. Liquid biopsy is a relatively noninvasive test that allows for repeated (longitudinal) sampling, enabling real-time tracking of tumor characteristics during treatment and thus monitoring temporal heterogeneity. Owing to this potential, liquid biopsy has emerged as a major topic in contemporary precision oncology research. The presence of various forms of tumor-derived cancer biomarkers in blood has been observed for a long time. Among the analytes used in liquid biopsy, circulating tumor cells were first reported in 1869 [2] as cells with tumor-like phenotypes present in peripheral blood, and in 1977, the existence of circulating tumor DNA (ctDNA) within cell-free DNA (cfDNA) in the peripheral blood of cancer patients was described [3]. More recently, it has been revealed that tumor-derived extracellular vesicles reflect the characteristics of their originating tumor cells, and they are now actively studied as circulating cancer biomarkers in blood. Today, liquid biopsy is understood not merely as a "replacement for tissue biopsy," but as a "translator of tumor signals" that reflects the patient's tumor status in real time.

1.4 Clinical Expansion and Future Outlook of Liquid Biopsy

The advancement of liquid biopsy technology is not solely the result of technical progress. It is the outcome of three converging factors: the development of highly sensitive molecular biology techniques, a deeper understanding of cancer biology, and the increasing clinical demand. Despite the long-standing observation of various tumor-derived markers in blood, the development of liquid biopsy methods utilizing these markers is relatively recent. This has been made possible by advances in molecular biology techniques capable of analyzing blood-borne tumor markers and by increased biological understanding of tumors over the past 10–20 years. It is the result of the interplay among advances in sensitive molecular techniques, deeper insights into cancer biology, and growing clinical needs. In particular, in 2016, the FDA approval of a liquid biopsy-based companion diagnostic for non-small cell lung cancer (NSCLC), which selects EGFR targeted therapeutics based on the measurement of epidermal growth factor receptor (EGFR) gene mutations in circulating tumor DNA (ctDNA) from patients, has marked a new milestone [4, 5]. Currently, liquid biopsy research is regarded not merely as an alternative to tissue biopsy, but as a tool that could redefine cancer diagnosis and treatment. In the context of early cancer detection, there is potential to identify ultra-early cancers that are undetectable by conventional imaging. For treatment monitoring, there is anticipation that molecular signals of recurrence can be detected much earlier than with imaging studies. Presently, liquid biopsy methods are being developed with the aim of expanding their application to various clinical scenarios, including cancer screening, monitoring of minimal residual disease after treatment, identification of treatment resistance upon recurrence, and treatment selection based on these findings. As of 2025, the FDA has approved numerous ctDNA-based companion diagnostic tests, and liquid biopsy-based MRD assays have begun to be incorporated into NCCN guidelines. Multiple global diagnostic companies are investing billions of dollars annually, demonstrating that liquid biopsy is transitioning from an experimental technology to a practical diagnostic tool. Moreover, liquid biopsy holds significant potential not only for clinicians but also for substantially improving patients' quality of life (QoL). If cancer status can be monitored through regular blood tests instead of repeated tissue biopsies, patients' physical pain and psychological burden can be dramatically reduced. Furthermore, liquid biopsy can serve as a big data platform for precision medicine. By accumulating tumor evolution data from numerous patients and integrating it with AI-based analyses, it becomes possible to design personalized treatment strategies on an entirely new level. However, it should be noted that, to date, liquid biopsy methods remain at a developmental stage; even those already FDA-approved and in clinical use do not fully replace traditional tissue-based biopsy methods, but are limited to providing complementary or additional information. Nevertheless, given the potential of liquid biopsy, it is essential for oncology professionals to understand its basic concepts and future directions for development. This book aims to explain the concepts of analytes used in liquid biopsy and their clinical applications and to introduce several liquid biopsy methods that are either FDA-approved and in use or currently under development (Fig. 1.2).

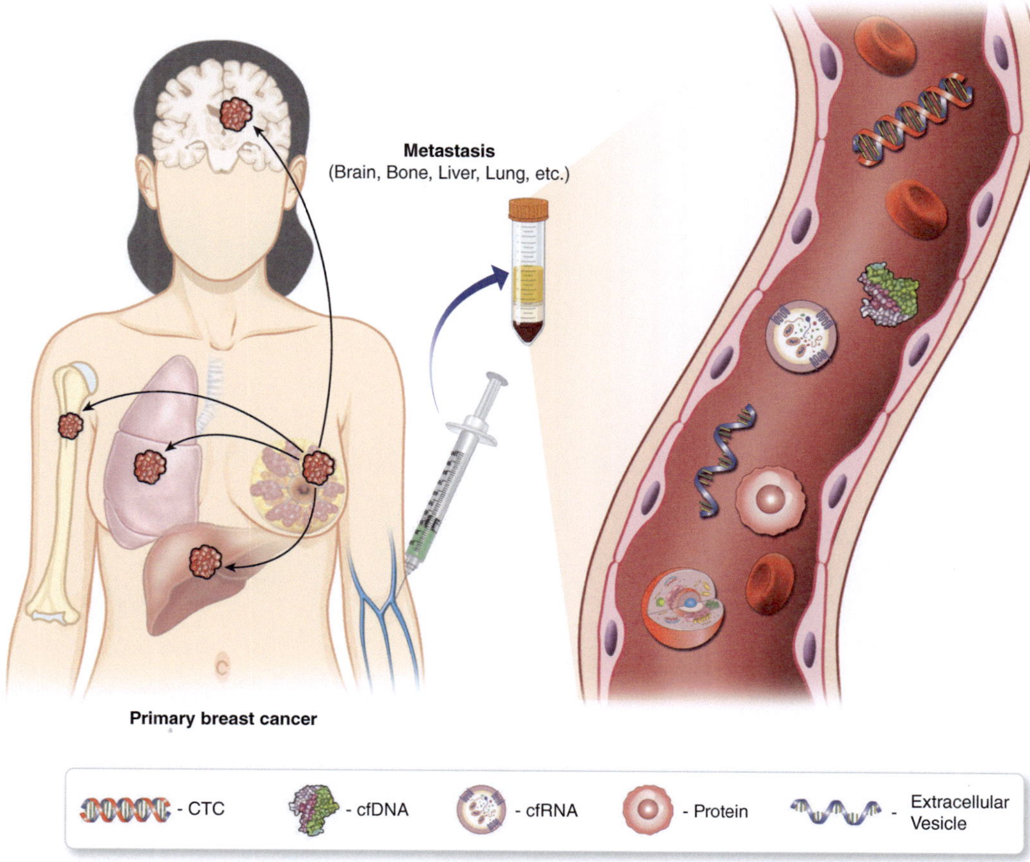

Fig. 1.2 Overview of breast cancer metastasis and liquid biopsy analytes

References

1. Heerink WJ, de Bock GH, de Jonge GJ, Groen HJM, Vliegenthart R, Oudkerk M. Complication rates of CT-guided transthoracic lung biopsy: meta-analysis. Eur Radiol. 2017;27(1):138–48.
2. Ashworth TR. A case of cancer in which cells similar to those in the tumours were seen in the blood after death. Med J Aust. 1869;14:146–7.
3. Leon SA, Shapiro B, Sklaroff DM, Yaros MJ. Free DNA in the serum of cancer patients and the effect of therapy. Cancer Res. 1977;37(3):646–50.
4. U.S. Food and Drug Administration. Premarket approval (PMA) [Internet]. [cited 2025 Apr 15]. Available from: https://www.accessdata.fda.gov/scripts/cdrh/cfdocs/cfpma/pma.cfm?id=P150047.
5. Thress KS, Brant R, Carr TH, Dearden S, Jenkins S, Brown H, et al. EGFR mutation detection in ctDNA from NSCLC patient plasma: a cross-platform comparison of leading technologies to support the clinical development of AZD9291. Lung Cancer. 2015;90(3):509–15.

Suggested Reading

McGranahan N, Swanton C. Clonal heterogeneity and tumor evolution: past, present, and the future. Cell. 2017;168(4):613–28.

Rao A, Barkley D, França GS, Yanai I. Exploring tissue architecture using spatial transcriptomics. Nature. 2021;596(7871):211–20.

Wan JCM, Massie C, Garcia-Corbacho J, Mouliere F, Brenton JD, Caldas C, et al. Liquid biopsies come of age: towards implementation of circulating tumour DNA. Nat Rev Cancer. 2017;17(4):223–38.

Biological Analytes in Liquid Biopsy

2

The analytes utilized in liquid biopsy are tumor-derived biomolecules present in blood and body fluids, comprehensively reflecting the genetic, transcriptomic, proteomic, and metabolomic information of tumors. The most well-known analytes include circulating tumor cells (CTCs), circulating tumor DNA (ctDNA), and extracellular vesicles (EVs), each providing tumor information at different levels—cellular, genetic fragment, and vesicular, respectively. In addition, several additional analytes have also been reported. For example, cell-free RNA (cfRNA), including mRNA, microRNA, and lncRNA, can reflect dynamic changes at the transcriptomic level. Tumor-educated platelets (TEPs), which are platelets with altered transcriptomic profiles due to tumor influence, have been proposed as unique biomarkers that can indirectly represent the status of cancer patients. Furthermore, blood proteins and metabolites, which have long been used in clinical practice, are also important components of liquid biopsy. Serum proteins such as alpha-fetoprotein (AFP), prostate-specific antigen (PSA), and cancer antigen-125 (CA-125) have been utilized in clinical diagnostics for decades, and recently, there have been active efforts to detect cancer cell-specific changes in energy metabolism pathways through metabolite profiling.

S. I. Kim, Y. Kim, *Liquid Biopsy for Cancer*, https://doi.org/10.1007/978-981-99-4418-7_2

As described above, liquid biopsy analytes provide multilayered information depending on their origin and characteristics. Circulating tumor cells (CTCs), as viable cellular units, contain the most comprehensive biological information, including DNA, RNA, proteins, and metabolites, and even allow for functional studies at the cellular level (such as ex vivo culture and drug response assays). In contrast, circulating tumor DNA (ctDNA), though present only in trace DNA fragments, enables highly sensitive detection of mutations, methylation, and structural variations, establishing itself as a key analyte for genome-based precision diagnostics. Extracellular vesicles (EVs), which are lipid bilayer vesicles secreted from cells, can stably carry nucleic acids, proteins, lipids, and metabolites, and are thus emerging as next-generation platforms for multimodal omics analysis.

Each analyte has distinct advantages and limitations (Table 2.1). For example, ctDNA, with its high sensitivity and standardized analytical methods, has seen the fastest clinical adoption, but it is limited in capturing protein expression or functional characteristics of tumor cells. CTCs are ideal for elucidating metastatic mechanisms and single-cell analyses, but their extremely low abundance in blood makes detection challenging. EVs stably preserve cargo that reflects the specificity of their cell of origin, but distinguishing between EVs derived from normal cells and those from tumor cells in the blood remains difficult.

Therefore, the future of liquid biopsy lies not in reliance on a single-analyte, but in multi-analyte integration encompassing CTCs, ctDNA, and EVs. Recent studies have sought to maximize diagnostic accuracy and predictive power by integrating information from different analytes. Indeed, some prospective clinical trials have reported improved surveillance of recurrence and prediction of therapeutic response by combining CTC enumeration, ctDNA mutation analysis, and EV miRNA profiling.

In this chapter, we focus on three analytes—CTCs, ctDNA, and EVs—that have either demonstrated clinical utility or are the subject of active research. We aim to compare and analyze their biological characteristics, clinical applicability, limitations, and future prospects.

Table 2.1 Advantages and disadvantages of liquid biopsy analytes for clinical application

Analyte		Description	Components	Advantages	Disadvantages	Applications
Tissue biopsy		Direct sampling of tumor tissue via surgical or needle biopsy	DNAs, RNAs, proteins, metabolites	Gold standard Identify the nature of cancer Rich molecular information Apply to various components	Invasive, risk of complications Hard to acquire continuously Higher heterogeneity depending on the sampling site Cannot reflect dynamic changes Very low abundance	Diagnosis Pathological grading/staging Classify molecular subtypes (e.g., IHC, FISH) Prognostication
Liquid biopsy	CTC (circulating tumor cells)	Intact tumor-derived cells circulating in the bloodstream	DNAs, RNAs, proteins, metabolites	Enable single-cell analysis Apply to various components Involve tumor-specific and intact molecules	Low concentration in the blood Heterogeneity across cells Technically challenging isolation Extremely rare event in early stages	Prognostication Drug resistance monitoring Metastasis mechanism studies (Predication)
	ctDNA (circulating tumor DNA)	Small fragments of DNA are released from tumor cells into the blood via apoptosis/necrosis	Double-strand DNA fragments	Highly specific mutation detection Quickly renewed Captures tumor burden dynamics Widely validated in clinical trials	Low concentration in the blood Mixed with normal cfDNA No spatial/phenotypic information Higher heterogeneity depending on clinical condition Low abundance in early tumors No cellular context May miss low-frequency clones	Prognostication Mutation profiling (e.g., EGFR, KRAS) Detection of MRD and recurrence Longitudinal treatment response
	EVs (extracellular vesicles)	Lipid bilayer-bound vesicles secreted by tumor and other cells into biofluids	DNAs, RNAs, proteins, metabolites	Protect biomolecules from degradation Reflect intercellular communication Abundant and stable in fluids Secreted continuously from cells Various components	Isolation and standardization are difficult Heterogeneous origin Undiscovered contents	Prognostication Biomarker discovery Possibility of diagnostic/prognostic panels Potential delivery vehicles Apply to multi-omics analysis

2.1 Circulating Tumor Cells (CTCs)

The possible presence of cancer cells in the bloodstream was first reported in the late nineteenth century. [1] observed cells in the blood during autopsy that were morphologically similar to tumor cells, providing the first evidence that cancer cells could be released into the circulation. However, for several decades, research on CTCs made little progress due to technical limitations and their extremely low frequency in blood. Until the mid-twentieth century, reports were largely limited to incidental morphological observations of tumor cells in blood smears. Interest in CTCs was renewed in the late 1990s with advances in isolation and detection technologies. In particular, the concept of "cell shedding"—the release of cells from primary or metastatic tumors into the bloodstream—became a key piece of evidence supporting the biological hypothesis of metastasis. As intact cells, CTCs integrate diverse biological information, including DNA, RNA, proteins, and metabolites, which is highly advantageous for detailed tumor characterization. However, for decades, the reliable isolation and analysis of the minute quantities of CTCs present in blood remained a formidable technical challenge.

Advances in cell isolation and molecular analysis technologies have marked a turning point in CTC research. The entry of CTC research into the clinical arena was catalyzed by the introduction of the CellSearch® system [2]. As a representative example of liquid biopsy technology that has achieved commercialization after extensive development, this platform isolates CTCs from blood using EpCAM antibody-based positive selection, followed by nuclear staining and fluorescence-based cell imaging. Tumor cells are quantified through analysis. CellSearch®, approved by the US FDA in 2004, became the first liquid biopsy diagnostic device used for prognostic assessment in patients with metastatic breast cancer. This marked the first instance of liquid biopsy being implemented in actual patient management beyond a mere research tool, representing a clinical turning point for CTC technology. CTCs are of particular analytical value because they are living cells. Unlike ctDNA, which only reveals DNA mutations, CTCs can simultaneously provide multilayered information, including DNA, RNA, proteins, and metabolites. This enables a comprehensive understanding of the tumor characteristics in each patient. For example, recent single-cell RNA-Seq studies have shown that CTCs in patients with metastatic cancer exhibit atypical activation of the Wnt signaling pathway, which has been identified as part of the mechanism underlying resistance to anti-androgen therapy [3]. Another study using whole-exome sequencing (WES) of CTCs from patients with metastatic prostate cancer discovered novel copy number alterations that were not detected by tissue biopsy, and these were directly associated with treatment response [4]. These findings suggest that single-cell analysis of CTCs can provide critical insights for designing personalized therapeutic strategies. Furthermore, CTCs serve as living evidence reflecting the spatial and temporal heterogeneity of tumors. As tumor cells enter the bloodstream, they undergo epithelial–mesenchymal transition (EMT), resulting in dynamic changes in cell surface markers, cytoskeleton, and motility. In particular, the co-expression of epithelial markers (EpCAM, CK) and mesenchymal markers (vimentin, N-cadherin) is important evidence of CTC plasticity, which is closely linked to metastatic potential [5]. Moreover, CTCs may exist as single cells or as clusters, known as circulating tumor microemboli (CTM). CTMs are notable for their higher survival rates in the bloodstream and greater metastatic potential compared to single CTCs [6]. Recent studies have revealed that platelets, fibroblasts, and immune cells circulate together with CTMs, contributing to the formation of the pre-metastatic niche. These biological discoveries indicate that CTCs are not merely "circulating cells" but can play an active role in the metastatic process. As illustrated in Fig. 2.1, circulating tumor cells arise through intravasation from the primary tumor and undergo a dynamic biological cascade that determines their survival, dormancy, or metastatic outgrowth (Fig. 2.1). From a technical

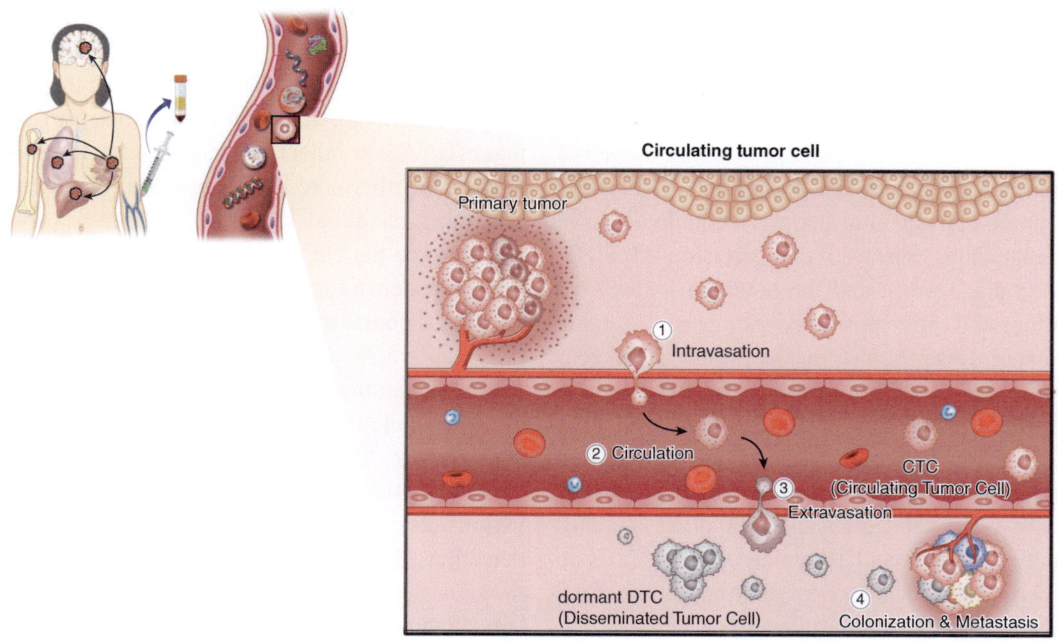

Fig. 2.1 Origin and biology of circulating tumor cells

perspective, because CTCs are based on living cells, they allow for a wide range of extended studies, such as post-analysis culture and drug response testing. In particular, the recent rapid advances in single-cell genomic analysis technologies have enabled the investigation of genetic mutations, copy number variations, fusion genes, and epigenetic modifications in CTCs. Thus, CTC analysis holds potential to contribute to various precision medicine decisions, including prediction of treatment response, detection of emerging resistant clones, and elucidation of metastatic mechanisms. Furthermore, recent efforts have focused on utilizing CTCs not just as biomarkers but as direct therapeutic targets. This involves isolating viable CTCs from a patient's blood and performing ex vivo chemosensitivity testing. By leveraging the unique characteristics of CTCs as mediators of metastasis, this strategy aims to identify the most effective drugs for a patient's cancer cells, offering substantial potential for providing practical information for personalized anticancer drug selection. However, there are several fundamental limitations to CTC-based analysis. The most prominent issue is the extremely low concentration of CTCs in the blood. Typically, there are only a few CTCs per milliliter of blood, and this ultra-rare presence poses an inherent limitation that is difficult to overcome, regardless of advances in high-sensitivity isolation technologies. Additionally, CTCs are a highly heterogeneous population both genetically and phenotypically, and some CTCs lose expression of epithelial markers (such as EpCAM) through the EMT (epithelial–mesenchymal transition) process. As a result, with conventional antibody-based isolation techniques, it is difficult to effectively detect these EMT-CTCs [7, 8].

Despite these limitations, a variety of non-antibody-based isolation technologies are being actively developed to overcome them. Representative examples include size-based microfilters, dielectrophoresis using electric fields, and microfluidic-based physical separation platforms [9]. These technologies offer the potential to capture diverse CTC subtypes while avoiding antibody dependency. Recently, artificial intelligence-based cell image analysis technologies have been introduced, greatly improving the automation and accuracy of CTC identification and quantification [10].

CTCs are the only "cellular" analyte among liquid biopsy analytes, and their ability to provide precise molecular biological information at the single cancer cell level makes them a powerful tool for real-time tracking of tumor evolution and metastatic potential. In particular, advances in single-cell genomic analysis technologies have dramatically improved the precision of CTC-based diagnostics, and the potential for ex vivo culture and drug sensitivity testing is also being realized. Nevertheless, due to technical and economic constraints such as the lack of analytical standardization, low detection rates, and high costs, CTCs have not yet been fully established as a routine clinical diagnostic platform. In the future, integrated analysis with other analytes such as ctDNA and EVs may enable CTCs to become a key component of multidimensional cancer diagnosis and prognosis prediction.

2.2 Circulating Tumor DNA (ctDNA)

The discovery that DNA fragments circulating in the blood are not merely remnants of dying cells, but also carry the genetic secrets of tumors, has significantly transformed the landscape of cancer diagnosis and therapeutic research. Circulating tumor DNA (ctDNA) serves as a noninvasive window into the genetic and epigenetic information of tumors, enabling real-time tracking of molecular events occurring within cancer patients.

To understand circulating tumor DNA (ctDNA), it is first necessary to define the concept of cell-free DNA (cfDNA). cfDNA refers to DNA fragments that are released from cells and freely circulate in the bloodstream, originating from normal physiological apoptosis or pathological necrosis. Such cfDNA is present at certain concentrations even in the blood of healthy individuals, and a portion of this is derived from tumor cells, which is referred to as circulating tumor DNA (ctDNA).

The origin of cfDNA has been observed for a long time. The existence of cfDNA was first reported in 1948, and in 1977, it was discovered that cfDNA could be detected in the plasma of cancer patients. Subsequently, [11] demonstrated that a portion of plasma cfDNA is tumor-derived, and [12] detected TP53 gene mutations in the urinary sediment of bladder cancer patients, proving that cfDNA can reflect the genetic mutations of tumors. Furthermore, [13] reported that gene mutations identified in tumor tissue were also found in the patient's plasma cfDNA, providing further evidence for the existence of ctDNA.

ctDNA contains tumor-specific genetic mutations, chromosomal rearrangements, and aberrant methylation, reflecting not only the presence of tumors but also their molecular characteristics and biological behavior. As a result, ctDNA is attracting attention as a valuable biomarker in various clinical contexts, including early cancer detection, monitoring of therapeutic response, prognosis prediction, and recurrence surveillance.

ctDNA is mainly released into the bloodstream during tumor cell apoptosis and necrosis, and in some cases, may also be generated by active secretion from living cells (Fig. 2.2). During apoptosis, DNA is cleaved into nucleosomal units (approximately 160–200 bp), which corresponds to the fragment size of cfDNA observed in blood. Therefore, the characteristic size distribution of cfDNA suggests that it results from apoptotic mechanisms, and ctDNA also follows this fragment structure. However, depending on the unique features of the tumor microenvironment, differences can be observed in fragment length, end motifs, and methylation patterns. These detailed characteristics provide important clues for distinguishing ctDNA from other cfDNA. In addition, cfDNA is unstable in the extracellular environment and is rapidly degraded. The half-life of cfDNA is relatively short, typically less than 2 h, and ctDNA is known to degrade even more rapidly [14]. ctDNA does more than indicate the presence of a tumor; it also reflects the biological behavior of cancer through tumor-specific gene mutations, structural variations, methylation abnormalities, and copy number alterations. As ctDNA can capture the genetic information and real-time changes of tumors, it is considered a key analyte for implementing precision medicine. In particular, ctDNA analysis is valued as a diagnos-

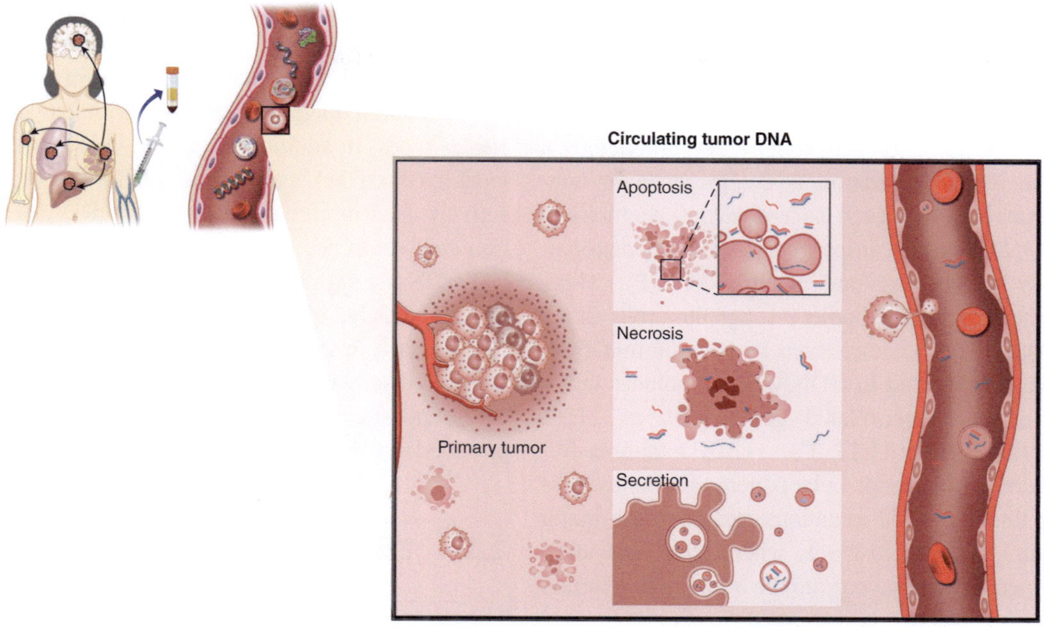

Fig. 2.2 Origin and biology of circulating tumor DNA

tic tool that can complement or, in some cases, replace traditional tissue biopsy, owing to its advantage of enabling repeated, noninvasive tracking of each patient's tumor genetics. It has a wide range of clinical applications, including monitoring treatment response, surveillance for recurrence, detection of resistance mutations, and companion diagnostics for drug selection. Its utility has been demonstrated in clinical trials, and its adoption in clinical practice is expanding. Furthermore, early detection of minimal residual disease (MRD) after treatment can contribute to identifying and monitoring patients at high risk of recurrence. Recently, ctDNA-based molecular diagnostic technologies are being actively developed as strategies for multi-cancer early detection (MCED). Beyond the detection of gene mutations, these approaches integrate high-dimensional molecular markers such as tumor tissue-specific genetic alterations, DNA methylation patterns, and cfDNA fragmentomics, enabling the simultaneous screening of multiple cancer types from a single blood sample with high sensitivity and specificity. Notably, these methods are gaining attention as promising diagnostic tools that can complement or even replace conventional imaging-based diagnostics, especially for cancers that are difficult to detect early (e.g., pancreatic, ovarian, and esophageal cancers). Their clinical utility has been evaluated and is being further assessed in large-scale prospective clinical trials such as the PATHFINDER trial, DETECT-A trial, and CCGA study. In the future, MCED technologies have the potential to fundamentally transform existing screening paradigms, and discussions are ongoing regarding their public health value and economic impact. Advances in ctDNA analysis technologies, including digital PCR (dPCR), BEAMing, and next-generation sequencing (NGS), have enabled the detection of extremely low levels of genetic mutations. As a result, ctDNA has become one of the most actively studied analytes in the field of liquid biopsy. However, despite technological progress, several technical and biological limitations remain. The first limitation is the extremely low abundance of ctDNA. Typically, the variant allele frequency (VAF) of ctDNA among cfDNA in blood is only a few percent or less, often below 0.1%, and in early-stage cancer patients, it can be reported as less than 0.01%. Such low concentrations often make detection challenging given current analytical capabilities, and the amount of ctDNA released varies greatly depending on biological factors such as tumor burden, lesion location, depth of invasion, and vascular distribution, posing inherent constraints on sensitivity and reproducibility. The second limitation is the presence of non-tumor cfDNA, which can reduce the specificity of ctDNA analysis. In particular, clonal hematopoiesis of indeterminate potential (CHIP), which arises from hematopoietic progenitor cells in the blood and is characterized by somatic mutations that are detected in cfDNA, often includes mutations in cancer-related genes such as TP53, DNMT3A, and TET2. These CHIP mutations frequently exhibit molecular patterns similar to those of tumor-derived mutations and can be a major cause of false positives, where ctDNA is interpreted as positive despite the absence of a tumor. In fact, CHIP is observed in approximately 10–20% of individuals over the age of 60, and it can serve as a significant risk factor for misdiagnosis, particularly in situations requiring ultra-sensitive ctDNA analysis, such as early cancer detection and minimal residual disease (MRD) monitoring. Various strategies have been proposed to overcome these limitations. Proactive filtering of CHIP-associated mutations through matched WBC sequencing, as well as analytical techniques based on the physical and epigenetic characteristics of cfDNA—such as fragment length distribution, end motif patterns, and key gene methylation profiles—are being introduced [15, 16]. Additionally, the adoption of artificial intelligence-based bioinformatics technologies enables the precise detection of subtle mutation signals within large-scale sequencing data and is being utilized for tumor-specific genomic profile matching and recurrence risk signature prediction. These technological advances are simultaneously improving the sensitivity and specificity of ctDNA analysis, thereby expanding its clinical applicability. Despite technical limitations, ctDNA is one of the most rapidly adopted analytes in clinical liquid biopsy and is utilized through various commercial products. For example, Guardant360® is a ctDNA-based gene panel test used to guide treatment decisions in patients with advanced solid tumors, capable of detecting key cancer-related gene mutations such as EGFR, KRAS, ALK, and BRAF. FoundationOne® Liquid CDx is also used to provide genetic information for companion diagnostics across a wide range of cancer types. In addition, Signatera™ is an individualized ctDNA monitoring platform that is actively used in clinical studies for MRD detection and recurrence surveillance. These commercial ctDNA assays are currently used not only in clinical trials but also as supplementary decision-making tools in some real-world clinical settings. Detailed discussion of these commercial technologies and specific clinical applications will be provided in the following section.

2.3 Extracellular Vesicles (EVs)

The observation of microscopic particles in blood dates back to the mid-twentieth century, making it relatively recent compared to other analytes. The existence of EVs was first reported in 1945 [17] as a "particulate fraction" during the isolation of blood coagulation factors, and in 1971 [18], it was confirmed that these particles possess a lipid bilayer structure and contain various proteins. At the time, they were considered merely cell debris or coagulation byproducts, but over time, the recognition grew that they are physiologically active entities secreted by cells. A pivotal turning point was the discovery that EVs possess immunological functions. In 1996, [19] first reported that B cell–derived exosomes are capable of antigen presentation, and in 1998, [20] demonstrated that dendritic cell–derived EVs could function as tumor vaccines. Together, these landmark studies established that EVs are not merely cellular debris but physiologically active entities with key roles in immune regulation. Since the mid-2000s, it has been revealed that EVs stably transport a variety of molecules, including microRNA, mRNA, DNA, and proteins, playing a central role in intercellular communication and microenvironment remodeling. As a result, EVs have attracted significant attention not only for maintaining physiological homeostasis but also as pathophysiological regulators in cancer, neurological diseases, and

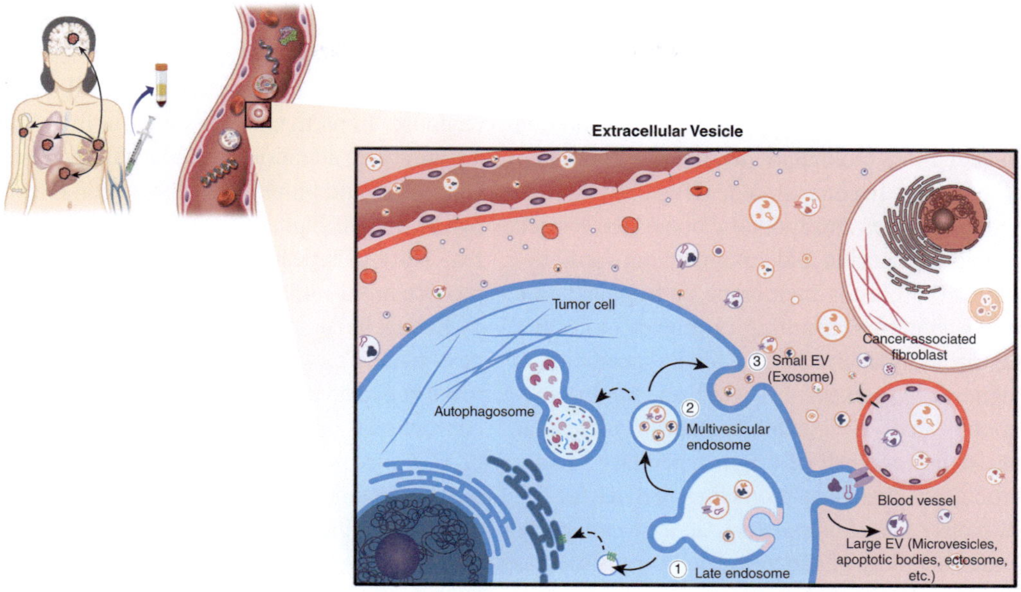

Fig. 2.3 Origin and biology of extracellular vesicles

immune disorders. In particular, blood-derived EVs offer the potential to capture diverse omics information—genomic, transcriptomic, proteomic, and metabolomic—through noninvasive approaches, highlighting their promise as precision diagnostic platforms (Fig. 2.3).

Extracellular vesicles (EVs) are lipid bilayer–enclosed particles secreted by cells mediating intercellular communication and transporting biomolecules. EVs are classified into various subtypes according to their size, biogenesis pathways, and biological functions. The main types include exosomes, microvesicles, and apoptotic bodies. Exosomes (30–150 nm) are formed as intraluminal vesicles within multivesicular bodies (MVBs) along the endosomal pathway and are released when these MVBs fuse with the plasma membrane, thus possessing an endosomal origin. During this process, EVs selectively encapsulate a variety of cargos—such as nucleic acids, proteins, and lipids—that reflect the biological state of the originating cell. When an endosomal origin is demonstrated, these vesicles are referred to as "exosomes;" more generally, they are described operationally as "small EVs." Microvesicles (100–1000 nm) are generated relatively directly and non-specifically through the outward budding of the plasma membrane, and they characteristically reflect the components of the plasma membrane from which they originate. Apoptotic bodies (500–2000 nm) are EVs released during the process of apoptosis, in which cellular components are packaged and expelled; these may contain organelles or nuclear material, resulting in the greatest structural heterogeneity among EVs. Recently, novel subtypes with unique sizes and functions beyond the traditional EV classification have been reported. For example, blebbisomes (up to 20 μm) are mega-EVs released from tumor or immune cells, exhibiting proteomic and organelle-level complexity and functioning as independent units [21]. Additionally, EV-associated nanoparticles such as exomeres, supermeres, and vault particles are being studied as new analytes that transmit complex protein/miRNA signals, and they display distinct differences from conventional small EVs in terms of size, density, and biochemical properties. Among these, small EVs of endosomal origin, typified by exosomes, are considered to have particularly high potential as diagnostic biomarkers due to the specificity of their biogenesis pathway. Small EVs undergo selective cargo loading during the formation of multivesicular bodies (MVBs) within the cell, and because these endosomal vesicles are released via fusion with the plasma membrane, they provide high-resolution molecular and biological information about their cell of origin. In contrast, other EV subtypes such as microvesicles and apoptotic bodies are formed through nonspecific and automatic outward budding of the plasma membrane or fragmentation during apoptosis, resulting in greater molecular heterogeneity and relatively lower specificity as diagnostic markers. Therefore, endosome-derived small EVs exhibit superior molecular consistency and cell-of-origin specificity and are particularly notable as promising analytes for liquid biopsy-based biomarkers, as they can stably contain a variety of cancer-related cargos such as miRNAs, tumor-specific proteins, and methylated DNA. The major cargos of these EVs include nucleic acids (DNA, mRNA, miRNA, lncRNA), proteins (membrane proteins, receptors, enzymes, etc.), lipids, and metabolites. These molecules are stably delivered via EVs and contribute to intercellular signaling, immune regulation, and microenvironment remodeling. Not only normal cells but also cancer cells actively secrete EVs. Tumor-derived extracellular vesicles (tEVs) from cancer cells can carry tumor-specific mutations in DNA/RNA and cancer-associated proteins. Normal and cancer cells differ in their genetic and transcriptional profiles at the molecular level, and these differences are reflected in the cargo content of their EVs. This distinction in EV cargo according to the cell of origin forms the basis for liquid biopsy approaches that utilize EVs for cancer diagnosis. In particular, tEVs can provide high-resolution molecular biological information about tumors, as they encapsulate multiple layers of genetic mutations, miRNA profiles, transcriptional regulators, and cancer-related proteins, making them valuable analytes for real-time monitoring of disease pathophysiology. Furthermore, EVs functionally participate in pathological processes—including tumor growth, angiogenesis, immune evasion, and formation of the pre-metastatic niche—underscoring their active roles beyond biomarker carriage.

Due to these characteristics, tEVs are considered a promising analyte with diverse clinical applications, including cancer diagnosis, prognosis prediction, and monitoring of therapeutic response. In particular, EVs present in the blood are attracting attention as an ideal biomarker platform for liquid biopsy-based precision medicine, owing to their high stability against degradation, feasibility of repeated sampling, and capacity to provide multi-omics information.

Extracellular vesicles (EVs) are emerging as next-generation precision diagnostic platforms that can overcome the informational limitations of conventional single-layer analytes such as ctDNA or CTC, as previously described, by simultaneously containing a variety of biological information—including genes, proteins, lipids, and metabolites—within a single-analyte. While ctDNA offers the advantage of sensitively capturing genetic mutations at the DNA level, it does not provide information on protein expression or functional status, and its fragmented DNA structure is prone to rapid degradation in the bloodstream, resulting in limited analytical stability. CTCs, although enabling cell-level analysis, are present at extremely low concentrations in the blood and have low isolation efficiency, and cells that have undergone epithelial-to-mesenchymal transition (EMT) are technically difficult to capture using conventional EpCAM-based technologies.

In contrast, tumor-derived EVs (tEVs) possess a lipid bilayer structure originating from cells, which effectively protects their internal cargo from extracellular enzymes, thereby exhibiting superior resistance to degradation and long-term stability compared to cfDNA or cfRNA. Indeed, it has been reported that EVs can retain analyzable nucleic acids and proteins even after cryopreservation, which is a significant advantage in terms of sample handling flexibility and clinical applicability.

Moreover, EVs can provide multilayered molecular information, including not only genetic mutations but also miRNAs, proteins, and metabolites, enabling their use as a multi-omics analysis platform that comprehensively reflects the molecular and functional characteristics of cancer. Notably, tumor-specific or cell-of-origin–specific markers (e.g., EpCAM on carcinoma-derived EVs) and EV-enriched tetraspanins (CD63, CD81, CD9), as well as integrins, can be displayed on EV surfaces, enabling selective enrichment and enhancing cancer specificity.

Although technical challenges remain, such as limited purification efficiency and a lack of standardization for tumor-specific EVs, as well as reproducibility issues across separation platforms, the development of high-purity isolation technologies combined with artificial intelligence-based multi-omics analysis algorithms is continuously improving the sensitivity and specificity of EV-based diagnostics [22].

In the future, EVs are expected to serve not only as standalone analytes but also as key components of integrated multi-analyte liquid biopsy strategies in combination with ctDNA and CTCs. Such integrated approaches are anticipated to provide higher diagnostic accuracy and clinical predictive power than single-analyte-based diagnostics, representing a significant turning point in the realization of precision medicine.

However, several technical challenges remain in EV analysis. First, EVs present in the blood are a mixture of those derived from normal and tumor cells, making the selective isolation of tumor-specific EVs difficult. To address this, immunoaffinity-based separation methods, size/density-based physical separation techniques, and microfluidic technologies are being developed and explored, but the establishment of high-purity isolation methods remains a critical challenge. Second, the heterogeneity of EV cargo and the lack of standardization across analytical platforms hinder the achievement of diagnostic sensitivity and reproducibility. In particular, standardization of pre-analytical conditions, storage duration, and purification methods is necessary to ensure the accuracy of various omics analyses, including miRNA, protein, and metabolite profiling.

For the implementation of precision medicine, liquid biopsy-based diagnostic methods must meet the following requirements. First, it is necessary to identify and validate cancer type-specific or patient-specific analytes. Second, clinical superiority in sensitivity and specificity—as compared with conventional imaging or single-marker assays—must be demonstrated. Third, prospective clinical trials are needed to evaluate whether liquid biopsy-based multi-omics diagnostics actually contribute to therapeutic decision-making. In this regard, EV technology remains at an early stage, and although its commercialization is somewhat slower compared to ctDNA, it holds significant potential to evolve into a next-generation precision diagnostic platform based on multiplexed analysis. A representative commercial diagnostic test based on EV analysis is ExoDx Prostate (IntelliScore, EPI). This test analyzes EV RNA extracted from the urine of patients suspected of having prostate cancer and is used to reduce unnecessary biopsies in patients with ambiguous pre-diagnostic PSA levels. It quantifies prostate cancer risk based on three mRNA biomarkers (ERG, PCA3, SPDEF) and is commercially available in the United States as a CLIA-certified test. Multiple clinical trials have demonstrated its high negative predictive value (NPV) and improved patient compliance. This example illustrates that EV-based liquid biopsy provides real clinical value in the cancer diagnostic process. The next section will discuss in greater detail representative cases of commercialized EV-based diagnostics and their current clinical applications.

References

1. Ashworth TR. A Case of Cancer in Which Cells Similar to Those in the Tumours Were Seen in the Blood after Death. The Medical Journal of Australia. 1869;14:146–7.
2. U.S. Food and Drug Administration. 510(k) Premarket notification [Internet]. [cited 2025 Apr 15]. Available from: https://www.accessdata.fda.gov/scripts/cdrh/cfdocs/cfpmn/pmn.cfm?ID=K103502.
3. Miyamoto DT, Zheng Y, Wittner BS, Lee RJ, Zhu H, Broderick KT, et al. RNA-Seq of single prostate CTCs implicates noncanonical Wnt signaling in antiandrogen resistance. Science. 2015;349(6254):1351–6.
4. Lohr JG, Adalsteinsson VA, Cibulskis K, Choudhury AD, Rosenberg M, Cruz-Gordillo P, et al. Whole-exome sequencing of circulating tumor cells provides a window into metastatic prostate cancer. Nat Biotechnol. 2014;32(5):479–84.

5. Yu M, Bardia A, Wittner BS, Stott SL, Smas ME, Ting DT, et al. Circulating breast tumor cells exhibit dynamic changes in epithelial and mesenchymal composition. Science. 2013;339(6119):580–4.
6. Zhang L, Ridgway LD, Wetzel MD, Ngo J, Yin W, Kumar D, et al. The identification and characterization of breast cancer CTCs competent for brain metastasis. Sci Transl Med. 2013;5(180):180ra48.
7. Carmona-Ule N, González-Conde M, Abuín C, Cueva JF, Palacios P, López-López R, et al. Short-term ex vivo culture of CTCs from advance breast cancer patients: clinical implications. Cancer. 2021;13(11):2668.
8. Kapeleris J, Kulasinghe A, Warkiani ME, Oleary C, Vela I, Leo P, et al. Ex vivo culture of circulating tumour cells derived from non-small cell lung cancer. Transl Lung Cancer Res. 2020;9(5):1795–809.
9. Ozkumur E, Shah AM, Ciciliano JC, Emmink BL, Miyamoto DT, Brachtel E, et al. Inertial focusing for tumor antigen–dependent and –independent sorting of rare circulating tumor cells. Sci Transl Med. 2013;5(179):179ra47.
10. Da Col G, Del Ben F, Bulfoni M, Turetta M, Gerratana L, Bertozzi S, et al. Image analysis of circulating tumor cells and leukocytes predicts survival and metastatic pattern in breast cancer patients. Front Oncol. 2022;10(12):725318.
11. Stroun M, Anker P, Maurice P, Lyautey J, Lederrey C, Beljanski M. Neoplastic characteristics of the DNA found in the plasma of cancer patients. Oncology. 1989;46(5):318–22.
12. Sidransky D, Von Eschenbach A, Tsai YC, Jones P, Summerhayes I, Marshall F, et al. Identification of p53 gene mutations in bladder cancers and urine samples. Science. 1991;252(5006):706–9.
13. Sorenson GD, Pribish DM, Valone FH, Memoli VA, Bzik DJ, Yao SL. Soluble normal and mutated DNA sequences from single-copy genes in human blood. Cancer Epidemiol Biomarkers Prev. 1994;3(1):67–71.
14. Cescon DW, Bratman SV, Chan SM, Siu LL. Circulating tumor DNA and liquid biopsy in oncology. Nat Cancer. 2020;1(3):276–90.
15. Razavi P, Li BT, Brown DN, Jung B, Hubbell E, Shen R, et al. High-intensity sequencing reveals the sources of plasma circulating cell-free DNA variants. Nat Med. 2019;25(12):1928–37.
16. Chan HT, Chin YM, Nakamura Y, Low SK. Clonal hematopoiesis in liquid biopsy: from biological noise to valuable clinical implications. Cancer. 2020;12(8):2277.
17. Chargaff E. Cell structure and the problem of blood coagulation. J Biol Chem. 1945;160(1):351–9.
18. Crawford N. The presence of contractile proteins in platelet microparticles isolated from human and animal platelet-free plasma. Br J Haematol. 1971;21(1):53–69.
19. Raposo G, Nijman HW, Stoorvogel W, Liejendekker R, Harding CV, Melief CJ, Geuze HJ. B lymphocytes secrete antigen-presenting vesicles. J Exp Med. 1996;183(3):1161–72. https://doi.org/10.1084/jem.183.3.1161. PMID: 8642258; PMCID: PMC2192324.
20. Zitvogel L, Regnault A, Lozier A, Wolfers J, Flament C, Tenza D, et al. Eradication of established murine tumors using a novel cell-free vaccine: dendritic cell derived exosomes. Nat Med. 1998;4(5):594–600.
21. Jeppesen DK, Sanchez ZC, Kelley NM, Hayes JB, Ambroise J, Koory EN, et al. Blebbisomes are large, organelle-rich extracellular vesicles with cell-like properties. Nat Cell Biol. 2025;27(3):438–48.
22. Welsh JA, Goberdhan DCI, O'Driscoll L, Buzas EI, Blenkiron C, Bussolati B, et al. Minimal information for studies of extracellular vesicles (MISEV2023): from basic to advanced approaches. J Extracell Vesicles. 2024;13(2):e12404.

Suggested Readings

Chen M, Zhao H. Next-generation sequencing in liquid biopsy: cancer screening and early detection. Hum Genomics. 2019;13(1):34.

Fernández-Lázaro D, García Hernández JL, García AC, Córdova Martínez A, Mielgo-Ayuso J, Cruz-Hernández JJ. Liquid biopsy as novel tool in precision medicine: origins, properties, identification and clinical perspective of cancer's biomarkers. Diagnostics. 2020;10(4):215.

Heitzer E, Haque IS, Roberts CES, Speicher MR. Current and future perspectives of liquid biopsies in genomics-driven oncology. Nat Rev Genet. 2019;20(2):71–88.

Siravegna G. How liquid biopsies can change clinical practice in oncology. Ann Oncol. 2019;30(10):1580.

Wan JCM, Massie C, Garcia-Corbacho J, Mouliere F, Brenton JD, Caldas C, et al. Liquid biopsies come of age: towards implementation of circulating tumour DNA. Nat Rev Cancer. 2017;17(4):223–38.

Pantel K, Alix-Panabières C. Liquid biopsy and minimal residual disease – latest advances and implications for cure. Nat Rev Clin Oncol. 2019;16(7):409–24.

Alix-Panabières C, Pantel K. Liquid biopsy: from discovery to clinical application. Cancer Discov. 2021;11(4):858–73.

Ignatiadis M, Sledge GW, Jeffrey SS. Liquid biopsy enters the clinic – implementation issues and future challenges. Nat Rev Clin Oncol. 2021;18(5):297–312.

Duffy MJ, Diamandis EP, Crown J. Circulating tumor DNA (ctDNA) as a pan-cancer screening test: is it finally on the horizon? Clin Chem Lab Med. 2021;59(8):1353–61.

Dang DK, Park BH. Circulating tumor DNA: current challenges for clinical utility. J Clin Invest. 2022;132(12):e154941.

Descamps L, Le Roy D, Deman AL. Microfluidic-based technologies for CTC isolation: a review of 10 years of intense efforts towards liquid biopsy. Int J Mol Sci. 2022;23(4):1981.

Couch Y, Buzàs EI, Di Vizio D, Gho YS, Harrison P, Hill AF, et al. A brief history of nearly EV-erything – the rise and rise of extracellular vesicles. J Extracell Vesicles. 2021;10(14):e12144.

van Niel G, D'Angelo G, Raposo G. Shedding light on the cell biology of extracellular vesicles. Nat Rev Mol Cell Biol. 2018;19(4):213–28.

Kalluri R, LeBleu VS. The biology, function, and biomedical applications of exosomes. Science. 2020;367(6478):eaau6977.

Jeppesen DK, Zhang Q, Franklin JL, Coffey RJ. Extracellular vesicles and nanoparticles: emerging complexities. Trends Cell Biol. 2023;33(8):667–81.

Konoshenko MY, Lekchnov EA, Vlassov AV, Laktionov PP. Isolation of extracellular vesicles: general methodologies and latest trends. Biomed Res Int. 2018;2018(1):8545347.

Yu DD, Wu Y, Shen HY, Lv MM, Chen WX, Zhang XH, et al. Exosomes in development, metastasis and drug resistance of breast cancer. Cancer Sci. 2015;106(8):959–64.

Pre-Analytical Considerations for Liquid Biopsy

3

Liquid biopsy, with its outstanding advantages of being noninvasive and allowing for repeated sampling, is already being utilized in various clinical studies as a tool to overcome the limitations of tissue biopsy. However, regardless of technological advances, analytical precision alone cannot establish liquid biopsy as a clinical standard. In fact, the establishment of pre-analytical processes optimized for each analyte is one of the decisive factors determining clinical applicability and is often an overlooked bottleneck in laboratory research.

Blood-based biospecimens are fundamentally different from fixed tissue. For example, tissue biopsies are stabilized through the formalin-fixed, paraffin-embedded (FFPE) process, which has been validated over decades. In contrast, blood is among the most dynamic and unstable biological environments in the body, with its composition subject to rapid changes within hours due to biological factors such as DNA fragment release from cell death, platelet activation, and hemolysis [1]. Therefore, every step from blood collection to the pre-analytical phase is not merely a matter of sample preparation, but serves as a key variable determining "clinical reproducibility."

In practice, liquid biopsy assays that demonstrated very high sensitivity and specificity in single-center studies have often shown suboptimal performance in multicenter clinical trials. A significant portion of this discrepancy can be attributed to subtle differences in pre-analytical procedures across institutions [2]. For example, one research group reported that a delay of more than 2 hours between blood collection and centrifugation resulted in a statistically significant decrease in ctDNA concentration, while another study highlighted that the type of anticoagulant used greatly affects CTC preservation rates [3]. In other words, these seemingly "minor differences," which may not significantly impact routine blood test results, can become critical variables for analytes such as CTCs, ctDNA, and EVs.

There is a wide range of variables that can affect the pre-analytical phase [4]. These include the type of collection tube (plasma vs. serum), choice of anticoagulant (EDTA, heparin, cfDNA stabilization tubes, etc.), delay time between collection and centrifugation, storage temperature and duration, whether two-step centrifugation is performed, handling of plasma aliquots, and the number of freeze-thaw cycles—all of which directly impact the sensitivity and specificity of the analysis [4]. Moreover, since EVs, ctDNA, and CTCs each have different biological stabilities and sensitivities, a single standard operating procedure (SOP) cannot provide optimal conditions for all analytes [2].

For this reason, international societies are making efforts toward standardization. For example, the ISLB (International Society of Liquid Biopsy), CANCER-ID consortium, and ISEV (International Society of Extracellular Vesicles) have proposed minimum standards for sample processing, storage, and reporting systems for

S. I. Kim, Y. Kim, *Liquid Biopsy for Cancer*, https://doi.org/10.1007/978-981-99-4418-7_3

each analyte, aiming to ensure consistency in multicenter studies. Although these recommendations are still evolving, they represent an ongoing effort to address the fundamental question of how to stabilize the complex and dynamic environment of blood. In clinical settings, it is particularly important to consider compatibility with real-world workflows, which differ from the stringent conditions of laboratory research. For example, while immediate two-step centrifugation after blood collection may be optimal for ensuring the sensitivity of ctDNA analysis, implementing this as a standard procedure in routine outpatient settings is challenging. Therefore, it is necessary to strike a balance between "technical excellence" and "clinical feasibility." If the analyte is inherently stable during pre-analytical processing, clinical implementation becomes relatively more straightforward. For liquid biopsy to expand as a core platform supporting precision medicine, it is essential not only to develop new analytical technologies but also to pursue scientific design and international standardization of pre-analytical steps. While advances in technology can improve analytical sensitivity and specificity, without systematic control of pre-analytical variables, clinical reproducibility and reliability cannot be guaranteed. Ultimately, pre-analytical considerations for each analyte will serve as a critical gateway to the "true clinical success of liquid biopsy" and will be among the most important factors in future large-scale multicenter clinical trials and regulatory approval processes [5, 6]. This chapter provides an in-depth discussion of the pre-analytical considerations required for each analyte—CTC, ctDNA, and EV—and systematically examines the challenges encountered in international standardization efforts and clinical implementation.

3.1 Circulating Tumor Cells (CTCs)

CTCs are cancer cells that have detached from the tumor and circulate in the bloodstream. Because they can be analyzed at the cellular level, they provide analyte information most closely resembling that of a tissue biopsy. However, as previously described, they are extremely rare and possess diverse physical and immunological characteristics, making their isolation and analysis challenging. Unlike ctDNA, which provides only fragmented genetic information, CTCs enable multidimensional analysis of tumor phenotype, transcriptome, proteome, and metabolome by allowing the direct capture of single cancer cells from blood. Nevertheless, CTCs are exceedingly scarce—typically fewer than 10 cells among 10^6–10^7 leukocytes in peripheral blood. Thus, isolating and analyzing CTCs is as challenging as "finding a needle in a haystack," where even minor variables in the pre-analytical phase can profoundly affect outcomes. The stability of CTCs declines rapidly from the moment of blood collection. When blood is collected in standard EDTA tubes, delays of more than 4 hours can result in cellular deformation and lysis, leading to damage of cell surface proteins and nucleic acid degradation. To address this, the CellSearch® system uses CellSave tubes to fix cell structures, enabling stable analysis within 96 hours. However, this process does not preserve the physiological functions of CTCs and imposes limitations on downstream analyses such as cell culture, protein function assays, and drug sensitivity testing. Recently, approaches to maintain the viability of CTCs have been explored [7]. Specialized preservation tubes without fixatives (such as Streck® and LBgard®) can ensure structural stability for over 72 hours while minimizing RNA and protein degradation [8]. However, these preservation technologies also affect other blood cells (leukocytes, platelets), which may increase background noise in subsequent isolation processes. Therefore, the choice of preservation method should be tailored to the intended purpose—whether for simple enumeration, single-cell genomic analysis, or functional culture studies. Three key pre-analytical variables determine the sensitivity and specificity of CTC analysis: the type of anticoagulant, centrifugation conditions, and storage/transport parameters. First is the type of anticoagulant used. Heparin can act as a PCR inhibitor and is therefore unsuitable for ctDNA analysis; it may also cause cell damage in CTC studies [9]. EDTA is the most widely used, but long-term storage can lead to cellular structural instability. Second are the centrifugation conditions. During plasma separation after low-speed centrifugation, cell loss may occur, whereas high-speed centrifugation can cause cell damage and fragmentation. Gradient centrifugation (such as Ficoll) is therefore employed, but this method has low efficiency in separating leukocytes and may miss some mesenchymal-like CTCs that have undergone EMT. Third are the conditions for sample storage and transport. Storage at 4 °C suppresses metabolic activity and increases stability for a certain period, but prolonged storage leads to cumulative cell membrane damage. Room temperature storage can cause rapid cell damage and senescence, although there are conflicting reports that some RNA profiles may actually remain stable. Therefore, optimization of pre-analytical conditions according to the analytical purpose is essential. To date, the only CTC analysis platform approved by the FDA is CellSearch®. This system features EpCAM-based immunomagnetic separation and a semi-automated enumeration process. CellSearch, when combined with the CellSave tube that ensures pre-analytical stability, allows for reliable analysis for at least 4 days. However, it cannot capture EpCAM-negative CTCs (cells that have undergone EMT) or mesenchymal-like CTCs, and because it includes a cell fixation step, functional studies on live cells are not possible. To address these limitations, recent studies have focused on the isolation of viable CTCs. Microfluidic-based platforms enable antigen-independent, label-free separation by exploiting physical properties such as size, electrical charge, and deformability, while maintaining cell viability. These technologies are being extended to ex vivo CTC culture, drug sensitivity testing, and single-cell RNA-seq/ATAC-seq, opening new possibilities for patient-tailored precision medicine. For example, some studies have generated patient-derived CTC organoids (CTC-derived organoids) from patient CTCs to directly assess anticancer drug responsiveness. This demonstrates that maintaining cell viability during pre-analytical processing is not merely a technical issue, but a prerequisite for the realization of precision medicine. In addition to single CTCs, circulating tumor microemboli (CTM, or CTC clusters) are also present in the bloodstream and are known to have 20–50 times higher metastatic potential than single CTCs. However, CTMs are relatively large and are easily destroyed during blood collection and centrifugation, making them susceptible to loss during pre-analytical processing. Recently, low-shear microfluidic technologies have been developed to preserve and isolate CTMs; however, standardized methods are still lacking. Therefore, the preservation of CTMs is one of the key pre-analytical variables that can affect the clinical predictive power of CTC-based diagnostics. Ultimately, CTC pre-analytical processing is not merely "cell storage," but a critical determinant of analytical sensitivity, specificity, reproducibility, and clinical interpretability. As technologies for isolating viable CTCs, preserving CTMs, and antigen-independent microfluidic platforms become more sophisticated, many pre-analytical limitations will be overcome. These advances will provide a crucial foundation for evolving CTCs from a simple "presence/absence" biomarker to a practical tool for patient-tailored precision oncology.

3.2 Circulating Tumor DNA (ctDNA)

Circulating tumor DNA (ctDNA) is an analyte with a very short half-life and is highly unstable, being structurally vulnerable to rapid degradation by nucleases in the bloodstream. As a result, every pre-analytical step from blood collection to DNA extraction influences analytical sensitivity, requiring rigorous control to ensure clinical accuracy. However, to date, no internationally standardized pre-analytical protocol exists, and significant heterogeneity remains between institutions in variables such as blood collection tube type, storage conditions, centrifugation methods, and transport times [10]. For ctDNA analysis, plasma is generally recommended over serum because during blood coagulation, a large amount of non-tumor cfDNA is released from leukocytes, which can dilute or contaminate the ctDNA signal. It is also essential to promptly remove blood cells by centrifugation under appropriate conditions within a certain time after blood collection, as this is a key procedure to minimize false-positive results caused by leukocyte-derived DNA [11]. In actual clinical settings, factors such as delays in sample transport, fluctuations in storage temperature, and limited equipment accessibility make it difficult to consistently control this process. Therefore, systematic management through standardized pre-analytical protocols is necessary. Although ctDNA is the most actively studied analyte in liquid biopsy, it paradoxically requires the most stringent pre-analytical control, creating a technical and operational gap that poses challenges for clinical implementation. The optimal blood volume required for testing has not yet been clearly standardized. In particular, in clinical scenarios such as early cancer detection or minimal residual disease (MRD) monitoring, where the variant allele frequency (VAF) is extremely low, the amount of blood collected can critically affect analytical sensitivity. Therefore, it is necessary to establish guidelines for appropriate blood collection volumes according to clinical purpose. The choice of blood collection tube is also a major variable. Since most analytical methods involve PCR-based amplification, EDTA-treated anticoagulant tubes are standard. In contrast, heparin-treated tubes can inhibit PCR reactions, and plasma obtained from such tubes may significantly reduce analytical sensitivity. Currently, commercially available blood collection tubes differ in composition and stability conditions depending on the manufacturer, making comparative studies and cross-validation between products essential in clinical practice. The Biorepositories and Biospecimen Research Branch of the U.S. National Cancer Institute (NCI) has issued the Biospecimen Evidence-Based Practices (BEBP) guidelines to enhance the reliability of cfDNA analysis. These guidelines specify detailed requirements for each step from blood collection to storage to maximize cfDNA quality and improve analytical sensitivity and reproducibility. First, during the blood collection step, the use of EDTA-containing anticoagulant tubes is recommended, and pre-chilling these tubes for at least 5 minutes prior to collection is suggested to help maintain cfDNA quality. The use of a 21–23-gauge butterfly needle is also recommended, as it minimizes cellular damage and reduces the release of leukocyte-derived cfDNA. The timing of plasma separation is critical for analytical sensitivity. According to the BEBP guidelines, centrifugation should be performed within 2 hours of blood collection. If unavoidable delays occur, centrifugation should be completed within 4 hours at room temperature (20–25 °C) or within 24 hours under refrigerated conditions (4 °C or 5 ± 3 °C) to help preserve cfDNA stability. However, such delays carry a risk of cfDNA quality degradation and should be minimized as much as possible. The first centrifugation is typically performed at 800–1600 g for 20 minutes at either 4 °C or room temperature, followed by a second high-speed centrifugation (14,000–16,000 g, 10–20 minutes, at room temperature or refrigerated) to remove residual cells or organelles from the plasma supernatant. This step is crucial for ensuring the purity of cfDNA suitable for analysis. Storage conditions directly impact the reliability of analytical results. Plasma obtained after the second centrifugation should be immediately stored at ultra-low temperatures (−80 °C). For temporary storage after the first centrifugation, plasma can be kept at 4 °C for up to 3 hours or at −20 °C for up to 3 months. It has been reported that storage at −80 °C can preserve samples for up to 9 months. Although isolated cfDNA has demonstrated stability for a certain period, even at −20 °C, a decrease in the number of amplifiable DNA copies has been observed during long-term storage. Currently, most researchers store isolated cfDNA at −20 °C; however, systematic studies on the effects of storage temperature and duration on cfDNA quality are lacking. Further validation is required.

Liquid biopsy-based diagnostics using ctDNA require not only precision in the pre-analytical process but also careful control of patient-specific physiological and biological factors. In particular, Clonal Hematopoiesis of Indeterminate Potential (CHIP), which is frequently observed in elderly patients, is considered a major factor that can cause false positives in ctDNA analysis.

CHIP refers to the clonal expansion of somatic mutations in hematopoietic stem and progenitor cells, commonly affecting cancer-related genes such as TP53, DNMT3A, and TET2. As a result, cancer-like genetic mutation signals may be detected in cfDNA even in the absence of malignancy. To exclude such effects, paired WBC sequencing, which involves simultaneous analysis of leukocyte DNA from collected blood samples, is necessary, and this requires appropriate pre-analytical processing [12, 13].

In addition to CHIP, various physiological and pathological conditions—such as the presence of benign tumors, tissue injury after intense exercise, lifestyle factors like smoking, and increased release of placenta-derived cfDNA during pregnancy—have been reported to affect the quantity and composition of cfDNA in blood. However, systematic studies on how these factors influence the sensitivity and specificity of ctDNA-based diagnostics remain insufficient.

Therefore, to ensure the accuracy of ctDNA interpretation, it is essential to recognize and control non-tumor-related factors that elevate cfDNA, implement WBC-based paired analysis strategies, and design appropriate pre-analytical procedures. Furthermore, large-scale prospective studies reflecting diverse clinical variables are needed.

3.3 Extracellular Vesicles (EVs)

Extracellular vesicles (EVs) are lipid bilayer–enclosed vesicles secreted by cells, and when present in blood, they serve as analytes that are relatively stable in the extracellular environment. The lipid bilayer protects internal cargo from various degrading enzymes such as RNases and DNases, allowing EVs to remain stable in circulation for longer periods compared to ctDNA or cfRNA. This property is one reason why EVs are considered less sensitive to pre-analytical variables.

However, there are still technical challenges to be addressed in the analytical implementation of EVs. Since EVs are released from diverse cellular origins, most commonly normal cells, tumor-derived EVs (tEVs) are estimated to account for less than 1% of the total. Therefore, selective enrichment of tEVs relevant to the analytical purpose is a key technological challenge.

Differential ultracentrifugation has been the most widely used method for EV isolation; however, this technique is heavily equipment-dependent, time-consuming, and carries the risk of reduced purity due to the co-isolation of similarly sized cellular debris or protein complexes. To overcome these limitations, methods such as size exclusion chromatography (SEC), immunoaffinity capture, and microfluidics-based technologies are being developed, but internationally standardized protocols are still lacking [14, 15, 16, 17].

In particular, immuno-based isolation methods utilizing EV surface markers (such as EpCAM, CD63, CD81, CD9, and integrins) are attracting attention as technologies that can enable selective enrichment of tumor-derived EVs (tEVs), thereby contributing to the achievement of high tumor specificity. However, most of these markers are not exclusive to tumor cells, as they are also expressed in normal cells. This cellular heterogeneity in expression complicates the consistency and reproducibility of analyses. For example, tetraspanin markers such as CD63, CD9, and CD81 are commonly expressed in nearly all EVs, limiting their utility for the selective isolation of tumor-specific EVs. Although EpCAM and integrin family markers have been reported to show relatively cancer cell-specific expression patterns, significant variability exists both among cancer types and between clones within the same tumor, which may compromise the target selectivity of immunoaffinity-based isolation methods. This biological heterogeneity can lead to reduced consistency across analytical platforms and decreased accuracy in clinical applications, necessitating complementary strategies such as multimodal approaches based on multiple markers or the integration of function-based isolation technologies. Considering these technical complexities and the sensitivity required during pre-analytical processing, the International Society for Extracellular Vesicles (ISEV) has recently issued key recommendations for EV analysis through the MISEV2023 (Minimal Information for Studies of Extracellular Vesicles) guidelines [18]. These guidelines provide minimum standards to enhance the reproducibility, comparability, and clinical applicability of EV-based research and include the following main points. First, the use of EDTA or citrate-based anticoagulants is recommended during blood collection and sample acquisition, and pre-processing should be performed as quickly as possible after collection to minimize hemolysis. Second, the choice of isolation method should be rationally determined according to the analytical purpose, with the advantages and disadvantages of each method—such as ultracentrifugation, size exclusion chromatography (SEC), and immuno-affinity capture—clearly described. Third, multi-layered characterization is required. Isolated EVs should be characterized based on various biomolecules, including surface proteins (marker proteins), lipid components, and RNA, and, where possible, quantitative and qualitative analyses should be performed at the single-EV (nanoscale resolution) level. A core aspect of MISEV2023 is the clear distinction between EVs and non-vesicular extracellular particles (NVEPs) according to the analytical objective. NVEPs include lipoproteins, protein complexes, and viral particles, all of which can confound EV cargo analysis. Therefore, the presence of NVEPs should be reported according to the analytical purpose, and the use of purity markers and negative controls in parallel is recommended to enhance the accuracy, specificity, and reproducibility of analyses. This is particularly critical in liquid biopsy applications targeting tumor-derived EVs (tEVs), as it underpins the preservation of cancer-specific signals and the prevention of false positives. In addition, various pre-analytical variables that affect EV preprocessing sensitivity—such as the type of anticoagulant, delay time after blood collection, storage temperature, presence of hemolysis or lipemia, and plasma viscosity—are factors that can substantially impact analytical results, necessitating the establishment of detailed criteria and standardization across laboratories [19]. In particular, for high-sensitivity analyses targeting low-abundance biomarkers such as miRNAs within EVs, prevention of cargo degradation, assurance of purity, and minimization of contamination are decisive factors that determine analytical reliability. These factors should not be regarded as mere experimental conditions, but as key variables directly linked to the accuracy and reproducibility of clinical interpretation. Ultimately, EV analysis is not a standardized process achievable through a single analytical method, but a high-precision molecular diagnostic platform requiring an integrated, end-to-end design encompassing collection, storage, isolation, purification, analysis, and interpretation. For the broader clinical adoption of EVs, international standardization of pre-analytical conditions for each analyte and the accumulation of validated data are essential. The EV preprocessing strategies presented in this chapter should be understood in organic connection with the clinical application cases discussed in subsequent chapters.

References

1. Gyorffy VJ, Dwivedi DJ, Liaw PC, Fox-Robichaud AE, Tsang JLY, Binnie A. Impact of sample processing delays on plasma markers of inflammation, chemotaxis, cell death, and blood coagulation. PLoS One. 2024;19(10):e0311921.
2. Batool SM, Hsia T, Beecroft A, Lewis B, Ekanayake E, Rosenfeld Y, et al. Extrinsic and intrinsic preanalytical variables affecting liquid biopsy in cancer. Cell Rep Med. 2023;4(10):101196.
3. Risberg B, Tsui DWY, Biggs H, Ruiz-Valdepenas Martin de Almagro A, Dawson SJ, Hodgkin C, et al. Effects of collection and processing procedures on plasma circulating cell-free DNA from cancer patients. J Mol Diagn JMD. 2018;20(6):883–92.
4. Peng H, Pan M, Zhou Z, Chen C, Xing X, Cheng S, et al. The impact of preanalytical variables on the analysis of cell-free DNA from blood and urine samples. Front Cell Dev Biol [Internet]. 2024 [cited 2025 Sep 5];12. Available from: https://www.frontiersin.org/journals/cell-and-developmental-biology/articles/10.3389/fcell.2024.1385041/full.
5. Danesi R, Lo YMD, Oellerich M, Beck J, Galbiati S, Re MD, et al. What do we need to obtain high quality circulating tumor DNA (ctDNA) for routine diagnostic test in oncology? – Considerations on pre-analytical aspects by the IFCC workgroup cfDNA. Clin Chim Acta. 2021;520:168–71.

6. Lee JS, Cho EH, Kim B, Hong J, Kim YG, Kim Y, et al. Clinical practice guideline for blood-based circulating tumor DNA assays. Ann Lab Med. 2024;44(3):195–209.
7. Qin J, Alt JR, Hunsley BA, Williams TL, Fernando MR. Stabilization of circulating tumor cells in blood using a collection device with a preservative reagent. Cancer Cell Int. 2014;14(1):23.
8. Grölz D, Hauch S, Schlumpberger M, Guenther K, Voss T, Sprenger-Haussels M, et al. Liquid biopsy preservation solutions for standardized pre-analytical workflows—venous whole blood and plasma. Curr Pathobiol Rep. 2018;6(4):275–86.
9. Yokota M, Tatsumi N, Nathalang O, Yamada T, Tsuda I. Effects of heparin on polymerase chain reaction for blood white cells. J Clin Lab Anal. 1999;13(3):133–40.
10. Kang Q, Henry NL, Paoletti C, Jiang H, Vats P, Chinnaiyan AM, et al. Comparative analysis of circulating tumor DNA stability In K3EDTA, Streck, and CellSave blood collection tubes. Clin Biochem. 2016;49(18):1354–60.
11. Kerachian MA, Azghandi M, Mozaffari-Jovin S, Thierry AR. Guidelines for pre-analytical conditions for assessing the methylation of circulating cell-free DNA. Clin Epigenetics. 2021;13(1):193.
12. Chan HT, Chin YM, Nakamura Y, Low SK. Clonal hematopoiesis in liquid biopsy: from biological noise to valuable clinical implications. Cancer. 2020;12(8):2277.
13. Gutierrez-Rodrigues F, Beerman I, Groarke EM, Patel BA, Spitofsky N, Dillon LW, et al. Utility of plasma cell-free DNA for *de novo* detection and quantification of clonal hematopoiesis. Haematologica. 2022;107(8):1815–26.
14. Théry C, Witwer KW, Aikawa E, Alcaraz MJ, Anderson JD, Andriantsitohaina R, et al. Minimal information for studies of extracellular vesicles 2018 (MISEV2018): a position statement of the International Society for Extracellular Vesicles and update of the MISEV2014 guidelines. J Extracell Vesicles. 2018;7(1):1535750.
15. Böing AN, van der Pol E, Grootemaat AE, Coumans FAW, Sturk A, Nieuwland R. Single-step isolation of extracellular vesicles by size-exclusion chromatography. J Extracell Vesicles. 2014;3:23430.
16. Livshits MA, Khomyakova E, Evtushenko EG, Lazarev VN, Kulemin NA, Semina SE, et al. Isolation of exosomes by differential centrifugation: theoretical analysis of a commonly used protocol. Sci Rep. 2015;5:17319.
17. Reátegui E, van der Vos KE, Lai CP, Zeinali M, Atai NA, Aldikacti B, et al. Engineered nanointerfaces for microfluidic isolation and molecular profiling of tumor-specific extracellular vesicles. Nat Commun. 2018;9(1):175.
18. Welsh JA, Goberdhan DCI, O'Driscoll L, Buzas EI, Blenkiron C, Bussolati B, et al. Minimal information for studies of extracellular vesicles (MISEV2023): from basic to advanced approaches. J Extracell Vesicles. 2024;13(2):e12404.
19. Lacroix R, Judicone C, Poncelet P, Robert S, Arnaud L, Sampol J, et al. Impact of pre-analytical parameters on the measurement of circulating microparticles: towards standardization of protocol. J Thromb Haemost JTH. 2012;10(3):437–46.

Suggested Reading

Payne K, Brooks JM, Taylor GS, Batis N, Noyvert B, Pan Y, et al. Immediate sample fixation increases circulating tumour cell (CTC) capture and preserves phenotype in head and neck squamous cell carcinoma: towards a standardised approach to microfluidic CTC biomarker discovery. Cancers. 2021;13(21):5519.

Kotikalapudi R, Patel RK. Comparative study of the influence of EDTA and sodium heparin on long term storage of cattle DNA. Cell J Yakhteh. 2015;17(1):181–6.

van Niel G, D'Angelo G, Raposo G. Shedding light on the cell biology of extracellular vesicles. Nat Rev Mol Cell Biol. 2018;19(4):213–28.

Kalluri R, LeBleu VS. The biology, function, and biomedical applications of exosomes. Science. 2020;367(6478):eaau6977.

Hoshino A, Costa-Silva B, Shen TL, Rodrigues G, Hashimoto A, Tesic Mark M, et al. Tumour exosome integrins determine organotropic metastasis. Nature. 2015;527(7578):329–35.

Coumans FAW, Brisson AR, Buzas EI, Dignat-George F, Drees EEE, El-Andaloussi S, et al. Methodological guidelines to study extracellular vesicles. Circ Res. 2017;120(10):1632–48.

4 Development and Validation of Liquid Biopsy Platforms

The advancement of cancer diagnostic technologies extends beyond the mere discovery of new biomarkers. To reach a level suitable for clinical application, it is essential to scientifically and systematically demonstrate that these biomarkers can contribute to actual patient diagnosis and therapeutic decision-making. This requires moving beyond simple "technical feasibility" at the laboratory level to establishing "clinical reliability" through reproducible data and rigorous clinical validation, enabling their adoption in medical practice.

The necessity for such evaluation became increasingly prominent in the early 2000s with the rapid development of genome-based technologies. Although numerous candidate biomarkers were reported, only a very limited number translated into actual clinical diagnostics. To address the so-called translation gap between research findings and clinical application, the Evaluation of Genomic Applications in Practice and Prevention (EGAPP) initiative under the U.S. CDC proposed a framework for evaluating genome-based diagnostic tests around 2007–2009 [1]. EGAPP's most significant contribution was the establishment of a structure that separates and sequentially verifies technical feasibility and clinical validity. This framework has since become the standard evaluation system not only for genomic diagnostics but also for emerging technologies such as liquid biopsy, companion diagnostics, and multi-omics platforms (Fig. 4.1).

1. *Analytical validity*—This stage assesses whether the biomarker can be measured accurately and precisely, both quantitatively and qualitatively. Key parameters include analytical sensitivity, specificity, reproducibility, and limit of detection.
2. *Clinical validity*—This stage demonstrates the association between the biomarker and a specific disease, as well as its diagnostic accuracy. It verifies how closely the biomarker is linked to the presence or status of the disease. This includes correlation with the disease, diagnostic accuracy (e.g., ROC curve, AUC), and prognostic predictive power.
3. *Clinical utility*—This stage evaluates whether the use of the biomarker leads to meaningful changes in clinical decision-making or improvements in patient outcomes. It demonstrates whether the adoption of the technology results in actual changes in patient management and, furthermore, contributes to improved patient outcomes such as increased survival rates or optimized treatment.

In the case of liquid biopsy, validation across these three stages is particularly critical. Analytes present in blood exist at extremely low concentrations, and sensitivity can vary greatly depending on pre-analytical conditions and analytical platforms. Therefore, merely demonstrating the technical feasibility of a biomarker is insufficient to obtain regulatory approval, and clinical implementation is even more challenging. In other words, establishing analytical validity does not

S. I. Kim, Y. Kim, *Liquid Biopsy for Cancer*, https://doi.org/10.1007/978-981-99-4418-7_4

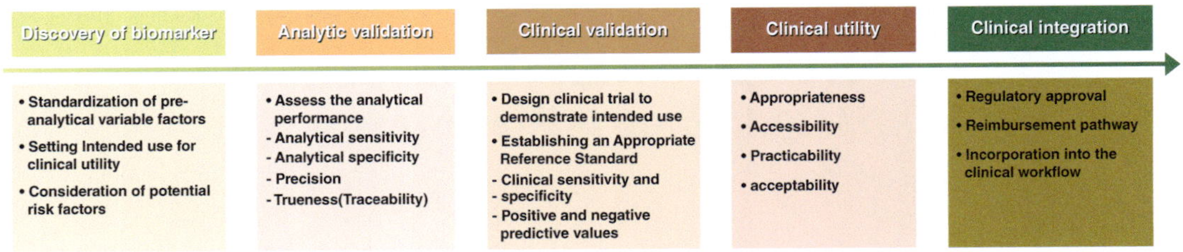

Fig. 4.1 Framework for biomarker assay development and clinical implementation

automatically guarantee clinical validity, and even if clinical validity is demonstrated, the technology cannot be implemented in actual clinical practice unless clinical utility—such as improvement in patient outcomes or cost-effectiveness—is also confirmed.

Moreover, these three pillars are closely linked to the core evaluation criteria of regulatory science. Regulatory agencies such as the U.S. FDA, EU-IVDR (In Vitro Diagnostic Regulation), and Korea's MFDS require evidence of analytical performance, clinical validity, and clinical utility during the approval process for new medical technologies. Therefore, for liquid biopsy technologies to progress beyond the research stage to global clinical trials, regulatory approval, and inclusion in clinical guidelines, it is essential to accumulate scientific evidence and validity data in accordance with the EGAPP framework.

Ultimately, this chapter does not merely enumerate theoretical concepts but rather explores, step by step, the process of gathering scientific evidence that demonstrates how liquid biopsy technologies transition *from laboratory experiments to clinical tools*. In particular, the distinct characteristics and limitations of analytes such as CTCs, ctDNA, and EVs present unique challenges during validation. In this chapter, we will conduct an in-depth examination of the development and clinical validation of liquid biopsy technologies, focusing on three key pillars: analytical validity, clinical validity, and clinical utility. These three stages are essential not only for technical validation but also for comprehensively assessing the potential for real-world clinical integration of diagnostic technologies. In particular, they provide the scientific and regulatory foundation necessary for the clinical adoption of emerging diagnostic technologies such as liquid biopsy.

4.1 Analytical Validity

Analytical validity refers to the ability of a specific assay to accurately and consistently detect and quantify a target analyte. This is a fundamental prerequisite for biomarker-based diagnostic tests to achieve clinical validity and clinical utility, and therefore must be rigorously validated from the early stages of assay development using quantitative and reproducible criteria. In liquid biopsy, where analytes are present in extremely low concentrations in the blood, establishing analytical validity is even more critical than in other molecular diagnostic technologies. For example, traditional tissue biopsies typically detect genes using more than several micrograms of DNA, whereas in liquid biopsy, it is common to obtain less than a few nanograms of ctDNA from a single patient's plasma sample. As a result, the limit of detection (LoD) and error suppression technologies become key indicators of the performance of liquid biopsy platforms [2]. Analytical sensitivity refers to the assay's ability to detect the lowest possible concentration of the analyte, and is generally characterized by indicators such as the limit of detection (LoD), limit of quantification (LoQ), limit of blank (LoB), and measurement range. In liquid biopsy, analytical sensitivity directly translates to clinical sensitivity, which is particularly crucial in scenarios such as early-stage cancer or minimal residual disease (MRD), where the variant allele frequency (VAF) is extremely low. For instance, Guardant360® utilizes a next-generation sequencing (NGS) platform with digital barcoding and error correction algorithms to detect variants at VAF levels as low as 0.1% [3]. Signatera™ employs a patient-specific PCR-based ctDNA tracking system, maximizing MRD detection sensitivity by tracking dozens of personalized variants selected from each patient's tumor tissue. Another platform, BEAMing (Beads, Emulsion, Amplification, Magnetics), is an ultra-sensitive dPCR-based technology that can theoretically detect variants at levels as low as 0.01%. The required sensitivity thresholds vary depending on the intended clinical application (early cancer detection, MRD, treatment response monitoring), and failure to meet these thresholds can lead directly to false-negative results. Analytical specificity assesses the potential for interference, cross-reactivity, and matrix effects from endogenous or exogenous nontarget substances that may affect the measurement of the target analyte. For example, blood from patients undergoing cancer therapy may contain chemotherapeutic agents or their metabolites, which can interfere with cfDNA purification efficiency or PCR amplification, potentially leading to false-negative or false-positive results in target variant detection. A representative case of analytical specificity assessment is the identification of CHIP (clonal hematopoiesis of indeterminate potential) as an endogenous interferent in ctDNA analysis. Mutations such as TP53, DNMT3A, and TET2, associated with aging or clonal hematopoietic expansion, have been reported to be misinterpreted as cancer-related mutations in ctDNA analysis, resulting in false positives, which can be particularly problematic in MRD detection. If a signal is detected due to CHIP in the absence of residual cancer, it may be incorrectly interpreted as evidence of residual disease, potentially causing significant issues in the course of treatment. Therefore, analytical specificity is no longer simply defined as "no cross-reactivity," but is being redefined in terms of the ability to distinguish and eliminate false-positive signals. To this end, matched WBC sequencing, fragmentomics, and methylation signature analyses are being used as supplementary indicators. Precision is an indicator of the consistency of analytical results and is divided into repeatability and reproducibility. Repeatability refers to the degree of agreement in results when the same sample is analyzed repeatedly under identical conditions (same operator, same equipment, single day). Reproducibility refers to the consistency of results across different operators, equipment, time intervals, or laboratories. For example, in the field of liquid biopsy, multi-center validation is often conducted according to the CLSI EP05-A2 guideline, and inter-laboratory tests using NIST reference materials are also performed. If, for instance, three analysts independently analyze the same ctDNA reference sample and the VAF results agree within ±10%, this is considered evidence of excellent precision. Precision is not merely an experimental metric; it is crucial for minimizing performance discrepancies in multi-center clinical trials and is directly linked to maintaining consistency between batches of equipment and reagents (QC/QA standards) [4]. Accuracy refers to how closely the analytical measurement approximates the true value or international reference standard and should be evaluated in conjunction with statistical uncertainty. Traceability assesses whether the analytical results are traceable to internationally recognized reference materials (such as those from NIST) or higher-order reference systems. For example, FoundationOne Liquid CDx verified both accuracy and traceability by comparison with standard gDNA reference materials provided by NIST in the United States. Liquid biopsy results are generally reported with quantitative values alongside confidence intervals or analytical uncertainty ranges, providing users with information on reliability based on concordance with the true value. Recently, NGS-based ctDNA panels are required to submit "concordance with reference standards" data for FDA approval. This process not only ensures technical accuracy but also serves as critical evidence for regulatory approval and insurance reimbursement. Analytical validity is not merely an auxiliary procedure for defining the specifications of liquid biopsy methods [5]. It is a fundamental process that provides key evidence supporting clinical performance, such as defining the reliable measurement range, determining drug compatibility and contraindications, and presenting confidence intervals for measured values. Therefore, it is essential to emphasize that analytical validity is a mandatory verification step that must be established from the early stages of diagnostic development through to final clinical application.

4.2 Clinical Validity

Clinical validity refers to the stage of evaluating whether a biomarker-based liquid biopsy shows a statistically significant correlation with disease presence, essentially verifying the diagnostic accuracy of the method—a key pillar in determining clinical applicability. Clinical validity assesses whether the method is appropriate for its intended use and can accurately identify patients in real-world settings. Therefore, its performance must be demonstrated through comparison with existing gold-standard reference diagnostic methods. Clinical validity is assessed using various statistical indicators. Clinical sensitivity refers to the proportion of actual patients who test positive, while clinical specificity refers to the proportion of individuals without the disease who test negative. Since clinical sensitivity and specificity are evaluated in subjects whose disease status is already known, retrospective studies are generally used. In this context, a clear definition of the gold-standard diagnostic method for determining disease status is essential. For example, demonstrating clinical validity requires that both case and control groups have their disease status confirmed by the same standard diagnostic method.

The positive predictive value (PPV) refers to the probability that a positive result truly indicates the presence of disease, while the negative predictive value (NPV) refers to the probability that a negative result truly indicates the absence of disease. PPV and NPV are likewise key indicators of clinical validity. However, PPV and NPV are calculated by comparing liquid biopsy results with the true disease status in patients whose condition is initially unknown. They are mainly evaluated in prospective studies. For example, in the PATHFINDER study of Galleri®, a multi-cancer early detection (MCED) test was prospectively evaluated in a general population at average risk [6]. The results showed a PPV of approximately 38% and an NPV of over 99%. This shows that screening tests may yield low PPV in low-prevalence populations but still provide highly reliable negative results (high NPV), supporting clinical utility. Additionally, concordance refers to the agreement rate (including positive and negative agreement rates) between biomarker-based analysis results and gold-standard results. For instance, in the PATHFINDER study of Galleri®, the liquid biopsy-based MCED test demonstrated over 90% concordance with tissue biopsy–confirmed diagnoses, thereby establishing its clinical validity [6].

The approach to establishing clinical validity varies depending on the intended use. In cancer screening, which targets low-prevalence populations, achieving high specificity and PPV is essential, and it is desirable to verify performance in the general population through prospective cohort studies. In this context, PPV and NPV are used as indicators of clinical validity. Since these are greatly influenced by disease prevalence, clinical trial design must consider the characteristics of the target population and the purpose of the analysis. For the purpose of aiding in diagnosis, it is common to evaluate clinical sensitivity and specificity by comparison with the existing gold standard.

Such clinical trials must be conducted with a sufficiently large sample size to ensure statistical power. In the early development stage, proof-of-concept can be established through pilot studies involving patient groups. However, for clinical application, large-scale prospective clinical trials based on representative populations that reflect the natural history and epidemiological characteristics of the disease are required. In particular, despite the advantage of being a noninvasive test, the greatest challenge for liquid biopsy remains achieving a meaningful PPV in low-prevalence populations.

Clinical validity is not limited to meeting numerical indicators such as sensitivity and specificity. It is crucial to demonstrate that the assay can maintain consistent performance across diverse populations, which is a key factor in determining external validity (generalizability). To this end, genetic and biological diversity must be considered. For example, not all individuals with the same genetic mutation will manifest the disease, a phenomenon known as penetrance. When a biomarker with low penetrance is used, clinical sensitivity may be overestimated. Furthermore, even among patients with the same mutation, there can be a wide spectrum of clinical manifestations, referred to as expressivity. In such cases, an assay sensitive only to specific phenotypes may fail to adequately capture the entire disease group.

In addition, differences in genotype frequencies among racial and regional groups also affect diagnostic performance. If a particular mutation is common in one ethnic group but rare in another, the corresponding biomarker may not be suitable as a universal diagnostic tool. Exogenous factors such as diet, environmental toxin exposure, and lifestyle habits also have a substantial impact on biomarker expression patterns and disease epidemiology. Ultimately, the key question is whether an assay can be effectively applied to diverse patient populations and whether its reliability is maintained under real-world epidemiological conditions. This serves as a criterion for determining how broadly the technology can be applied in actual clinical settings and ultimately forms the foundation for assessing the diagnostic reliability and clinical integration potential of liquid biopsy technologies. In summary, it is important to remember that clinical validity does not end with simply meeting statistical indicators of the clinical performance of an assay. Rather, it should be understood as the process of demonstrating that a given biomarker can accurately identify patients in real-world clinical environments and maintain consistent performance across diverse populations and epidemiological conditions. While metrics such as sensitivity, specificity, PPV, NPV, and concordance are essential, true clinical validity is achieved when these figures adequately reflect the biological diversity of patient populations and the natural history of disease. Thus, liquid biopsy must demonstrate generalizability through large-scale prospective trials and diverse population studies to be established as a reliable clinical tool. This is an essential gateway for liquid biopsy technologies to move beyond laboratory discoveries and into real-world clinical applications in precision oncology.

4.3 Clinical Utility

Clinical utility refers to the evaluation of whether a diagnostic test produces meaningful changes in patient management, prognosis prediction, or disease monitoring in clinical practice [7]. This goes beyond merely providing information about biomarkers or genetic variants; it involves demonstrating that the test results influence clinical decision-making, ultimately leading to improvements in patient quality of life, survival rates, and optimization of healthcare resources. The core of clinical utility lies not in the "provision of information," but in the "change in action." Therefore, it is necessary to assess whether the test results have led to actual clinical interventions. Specific examples include ① modification of treatment strategies, ② adjustment of monitoring intervals or methods, ③ omission of unnecessary tissue biopsies or additional diagnostic procedures, and ④ early inclusion in or exclusion from specific therapies. Such changes in clinical practice must be supported by patient-centered clinical benefits, and potential risks such as overdiagnosis or overtreatment should also be considered alongside potential benefits. Accordingly, the evaluation of clinical utility must address the following key questions:

- Did the test results lead to actual changes in treatment?
- Was cost-effectiveness improved compared to existing diagnostic methods?
- Did the test enable early diagnosis or prevent inappropriate treatment?
- Did it help prevent overdiagnosis or overtreatment?

Representative examples demonstrating clinical utility include the MSK-IMPACT and MSK-ACCESS platforms developed at Memorial Sloan Kettering Cancer Center [8]. MSK-IMPACT, the first comprehensive tumor gene panel test approved by the FDA in 2017, can analyze up to 468 cancer-related genes for somatic mutations as well as microsatellite instability (MSI) and tumor mutational burden (TMB). This assay has led to substantial changes in treatment selection for cancer patients. For example, immune checkpoint inhibitors were administered to patients with MSI-H or high TMB, and patients with identified driver mutations gained access to targeted therapies, enabling new treatment strategies for patient groups with limited options under conventional therapies. Additionally, by simultaneously detecting multiple mutations in a single panel test rather than performing repeated single-gene assays, cost-effectiveness was improved, and unnecessary chemotherapy could be avoided or alternative treatments applied early in patients with rare subtypes. At the same time, variants of uncertain clinical significance (VUS) were reported but not considered in treatment decisions, thereby reducing the risk of overtreatment. In this way, MSK-IMPACT serves as a representative example of how analysis results can directly influence therapeutic strategies and optimize the use of clinical resources. Subsequently, MSK-ACCESS was developed as a liquid biopsy-based cfDNA analysis platform, providing high-depth analysis of 129 genes validated by MSK-IMPACT. This technology enables the noninvasive detection of actionable mutations even in patients for whom tissue biopsy is not feasible or repeated procedures are risky, thereby greatly improving access to targeted therapies. Furthermore, it allows for early detection of clonal evolution or drug resistance mutations during treatment, enabling timely adjustment of therapeutic strategies before clinical deterioration occurs. Notably, the inclusion of matched WBC sequencing to filter out CHIP (clonal hematopoiesis)-derived variants helps prevent unnecessary therapeutic interventions due to false positives. The blood-based approach also facilitates longitudinal monitoring in the same patient, allowing for efficient assessment of recurrence risk and monitoring of treatment response. These features reduce the costs and complications associated with repeated tissue biopsies and enhance the efficient use of healthcare resources. Ultimately, the experiences with MSK-IMPACT and MSK-ACCESS clearly illustrate the concept of clinical utility. These platforms are not merely tools for providing molecular information; they have brought about changes across patient management, including modification of therapeutic strategies, improved cost-effectiveness, prevention of inappropriate treatments, and avoidance of unnecessary procedures. This serves as a representative example demonstrating that clinical utility extends beyond "analytical accuracy" to encompass "improvement in patient outcomes and changes in clinical practice." Therefore, establishing clinical utility is the final critical step for liquid biopsy technologies to move beyond laboratory discovery and become practical tools in precision oncology [9].

References

1. Teutsch SM, Bradley LA, Palomaki GE, Haddow JE, Piper M, Calonge N, Dotson WD, Douglas MP, Berg AO, EGAPP Working Group. The evaluation of genomic applications in practice and prevention (EGAPP) initiative: methods of the EGAPP Working Group. Genet Med. 2009;11(1):3–14. https://doi.org/10.1097/GIM.0b013e318184137c. PMID: 18813139; PMCID: PMC2743609.
2. Lanman RB, Mortimer SA, Zill OA, Sebisanovic D, Lopez R, Blau S, et al. Analytical and clinical validation of a digital sequencing panel for quantitative, highly accurate evaluation of cell-free circulating tumor DNA. PLoS One. 2015;10(10):e0140712.
3. Bauml JM, Li BT, Velcheti V, Govindan R, Curioni-Fontecedro A, Dooms C, Takahashi T, Duda AW, Odegaard JI, Cruz-Guilloty F, Jin L, Zhang Y, Anderson A, Skoulidis F. Clinical validation of Guardant360 CDx as a blood-based companion diagnostic for sotorasib. Lung Cancer. 2022;166:270–8. https://doi.org/10.1016/j.lungcan.2021.10.007. Epub 2021 Oct 19. PMID: 34838325; PMCID: PMC10325630.
4. Stetson D, Ahmed A, Xu X, Nuttall BRB, Lubinski TJ, Johnson JH, et al. Orthogonal comparison of four plasma NGS tests with tumor suggests technical factors are a major source of assay discordance. JCO Precis Oncol. 2019;3:1–9.

5. Merker JD, Oxnard GR, Compton C, Diehn M, Hurley P, Lazar AJ, et al. Circulating tumor DNA analysis in patients with cancer: American Society of Clinical Oncology and College of American Pathologists Joint Review. J Clin Oncol [Internet]. 2018 [cited 2025 Apr 29]. Available from: https://ascopubs.org/doi/10.1200/JCO.2017.76.8671.
6. Schrag D, Beer TM, McDonnell CH, Nadauld L, Dilaveri CA, Reid R, et al. Blood-based tests for multicancer early detection (PATHFINDER): a prospective cohort study. Lancet. 2023;402(10409):1251–60.
7. Hayes DF, Bast RC, Desch CE, Fritsche H Jr, Kemeny NE, Jessup JM, Locker GY, Macdonald JS, Mennel RG, Norton L, et al. Defining clinical utility of tumor biomarker tests: a clinician's view. J Clin Oncol. 2021;39(3):238–48.
8. U.S. Food and Drug Administration. Evaluation of automatic Class III designation for MSK-IMPACT (DEN170058). FDA Decision Summary. 2017. Available at: https://www.accessdata.fda.gov/cdrh_docs/reviews/den170058.pdf.
9. Goodsaid FM, Mendrick DL. The labyrinth of product development and regulatory science: cfDNA liquid biopsies at the FDA. Clin Transl Sci. 2019;12(5):421–7.

Suggested Readings

Siravegna G. How liquid biopsies can change clinical practice in oncology. Ann Oncol. 2019;30(10):1580.

Clinical and Laboratory Standards Institute (CLSI). Evaluation of precision of quantitative measurement procedures; approved guideline—third edition (EP05-A3). Wayne: CLSI; 2014.

Clinical and Laboratory Standards Institute (CLSI). Evaluation of the linearity of quantitative measurement procedures: a statistical approach (EP06-A). Wayne: CLSI; 2003.

Clinical and Laboratory Standards Institute (CLSI). Interference testing in clinical chemistry; approved guideline—second edition (EP07-A2). Wayne: CLSI; 2005.

Clinical and Laboratory Standards Institute (CLSI). Evaluation of detection capability for clinical laboratory measurement procedures; approved guideline—second edition (EP17-A2). Wayne: CLSI; 2012.

Clinical and Laboratory Standards Institute (CLSI). Verification and validation of multiplex nucleic acid assays (MM17-A). Wayne: CLSI; 2008.

Clinical and Laboratory Standards Institute (CLSI). Nucleic acid sequencing methods in diagnostic laboratory medicine; approved guideline—second edition (MM09-A2). Wayne: CLSI; 2014.

Global Harmonization Task Force (GHTF). Clinical evidence for IVD medical devices – key definitions and concepts (SG5/N7:2012). GHTF; 2012.

Global Harmonization Task Force (GHTF). Clinical performance studies for in vitro diagnostic medical devices (SG5/N8:2012). GHTF; 2012.

International Medical Device Regulators Forum (IMDRF). In: Principles of clinical evidence for in vitro diagnostic medical devices (IVD WG/N52:2017). IMDRF; 2017.

5 Clinical Applications of Liquid Biopsy

The Figure 5.1 above visually arranges the entire process of cancer diagnosis and treatment along a timeline, illustrating the clinical scenarios in which liquid biopsy can be utilized. The greatest strengths of liquid biopsy are its noninvasiveness and the ability for repeated sampling. Unlike single-point tissue biopsies, this enables continuous tracking of molecular changes in the tumor, clearly distinguishing it from conventional imaging or tissue-based diagnostic methods. This repeatability enables tracking of dynamic biological events—such as tumor burden changes, recurrence, clonal evolution, MRD, and resistance—rather than offering only a static snapshot. As a result, liquid biopsy can serve as a complementary or alternative approach to capture dynamic tumor evolution, which is often missed by traditional diagnostic strategies based on a single, fixed tissue sample. In practice, genetic discordance between primary and metastatic sites is frequently observed in metastatic cancer, and tissue biopsy is often limited by anatomical constraints, making it unlikely to represent the entire disease status [1, 2]. Liquid biopsy is increasingly recognized as a clinical strategy to overcome these limitations. Currently, the most widely used liquid biopsy technology in clinical practice is ctDNA-based analysis [3–5]. It is broadly applied in monitoring treatment response, companion diagnostics, and detection of resistance mutations in metastatic solid tumors, with several applications already approved by the FDA [3]. For example, detecting the T790M resistance mutation in ctDNA after EGFR-targeted therapy and using this information to guide subsequent treatment selection demonstrates that liquid biopsy can contribute directly to clinical decision-making, beyond its role as a research tool [6]. Recently, the clinical utility of ctDNA has expanded to include cancer screening, MRD monitoring, and surveillance during asymptomatic periods, covering the entire clinical continuum before and after treatment [7–10]. At the same time, liquid biopsy technologies based on various analytes—such as exosomal nucleic acids, cancer-specific miRNAs, tumor-derived proteins, and DNA methylation patterns—are also being actively developed. They are being developed in parallel, with some already showing significant clinical results.

As such, liquid biopsy is gaining attention as a powerful tool that can address several limitations of tissue biopsy for clinical implementation. However, there are also important limitations that must not be overlooked in its interpretation. All circulating biomarkers analyzed in liquid biopsy are obtained from blood, an indirect environment rather than tissue, and the biological information derived from them should be interpreted as a "high-probability inference" regarding their potential tumor origin. For example, while ctDNA, EVs, and CTCs can all reflect tumor-derived characteristics, their secretion mechanisms are not fully elucidated, and similar molecules may in fact be secreted from non-tumor tissues as well [11, 12]. In particular, since

S. I. Kim, Y. Kim, *Liquid Biopsy for Cancer*, https://doi.org/10.1007/978-981-99-4418-7_5

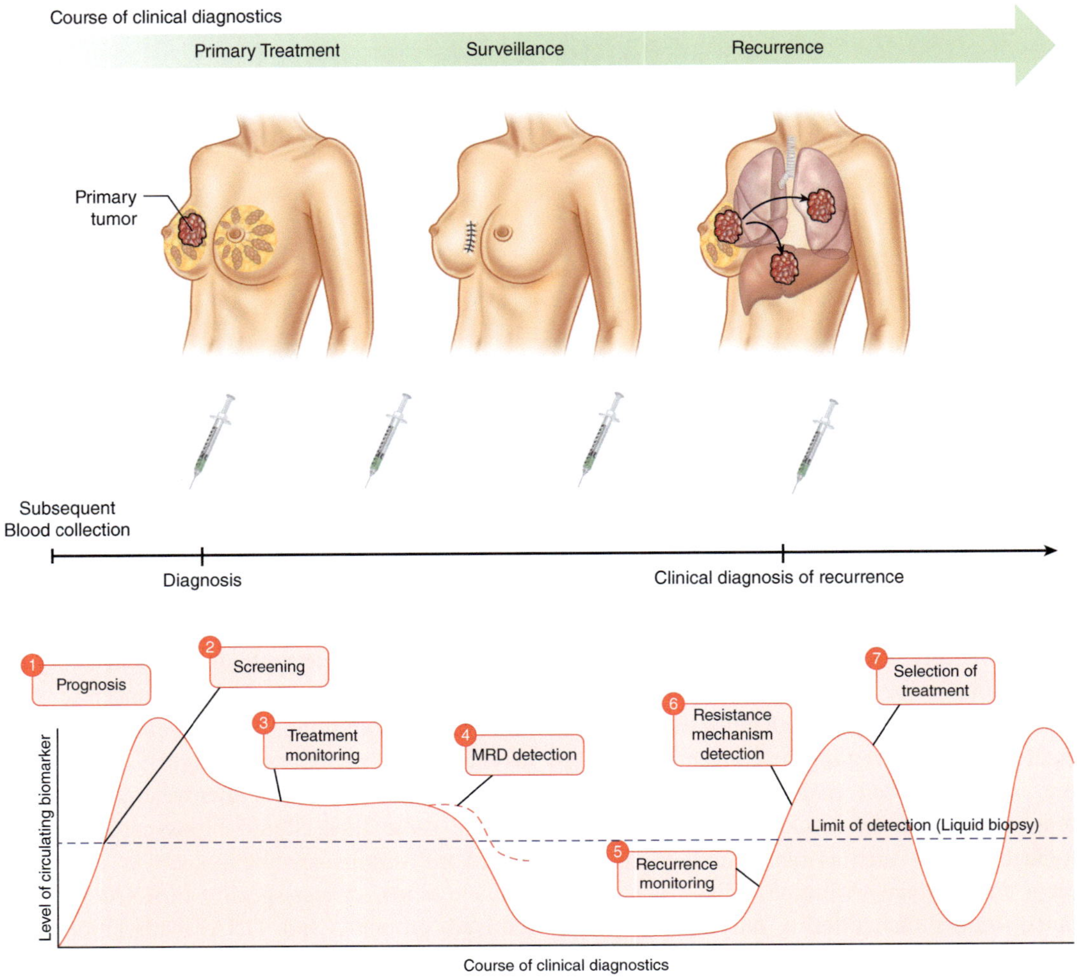

Fig. 5.1 Clinical application of liquid biopsy across the cancer care continuum

the circulatory system contains not only immune cells, inflammatory cells, and blood cells, but also cells and cell fragments originating from various organs, "tumor specificity" must always be rigorously validated as a core criterion in analysis [3, 11].

Therefore, improving sensitivity alone is insufficient; robust biological and technical evidence confirming the tumor origin of biomarkers is also required. In other words, can the biomarker be sufficiently distinguished from nonspecific or non-tumor signals? Can analytical accuracy and consistency be ensured? And, based on this, can it objectively be demonstrated to influence clinical decision-making? Such validation is essential. This is why a comprehensive performance evaluation of analytical validity, clinical validity, and clinical utility is required [3].

In particular, for liquid biopsy technologies to be used in real-world clinical settings, it is essential to clearly define the intended purpose of the technology. This is not merely a matter of technical application, but rather, the "intended use"—that is, "which clinical question is being addressed in which patient population?"—forms the foundation for assay evaluation. For example, whether the technology is for cancer screening, as an adjunct tool for monitoring treatment response, or as a companion diagnostic for therapy selection, the required standards for sensitivity, specificity, and predictive value will inevitably differ. Therefore, designing the assay according to its intended use and demonstrating performance that meets those requirements is key not only to development but also to establishing the scientific validity and regulatory acceptability of clinical implementation.

Ultimately, rather than making definitive diagnoses based on a single marker or analyte, liquid biopsy should evolve toward enhancing interpretive precision and reliability through comprehensive pattern analysis, multi-omics integration, and repeated longitudinal sampling. Recognizing this approach actually strengthens the scientific utility of liquid biopsy.

In this chapter, we will examine the clinical applications of liquid biopsy according to intended use scenarios, categorized into the following four areas:

- Cancer Screening (Early Cancer Detection)
- Minimal Residual Disease (MRD) Detection and Recurrence Monitoring
- Companion Diagnostics
- Detection of Resistance Mutations

In each scenario, we will examine not only the selection of analytes and technical implementation but also simultaneously assess the possibilities and limitations within the three pillars of analytical validity, clinical validity, and clinical utility. This framework will serve to explore the scientific evidence and clinical rationale for whether liquid biopsy can complement or ultimately replace existing diagnostic technologies in certain domains.

5.1 Early Cancer Detection and Screening

Early cancer detection is considered one of the most effective strategies for improving patient survival rates and reducing the burden of treatment. In particular, since most solid tumors are diagnosed at an advanced stage when symptoms appear, the ability to detect cancer-specific biomarkers during the asymptomatic phase could fundamentally change the paradigm of diagnosis and treatment. Recent studies have revealed that cancer cell-derived DNA, RNA, proteins, and extracellular vesicles (EVs) are released into blood and other body fluids even at the earliest stages of disease. As a result, blood-based liquid biopsy has attracted attention as a promising tool for early diagnosis.

It is essential to distinguish between the concepts of "early detection" and "screening." Early detection refers to identifying cancer as early as possible before symptoms develop, in individuals with suspicious findings on conventional diagnostic or imaging tests, or those with genetic risk factors or a family history of cancer. In contrast, screening is a public health approach aimed at selectively identifying the presence or absence of cancer in asymptomatic individuals from the general population with average risk (Fig. 5.2). These two approaches differ in clinical trial design, performance evaluation metrics, and regulatory strategies. Screening, in particular, is regarded as a public health intervention, and thus, in addition to sensitivity and specificity, positive predictive value (PPV), negative predictive value (NPV), cost-benefit balance, risk of overdiagnosis or overtreatment, and the potential for protocol simplification must all be considered [3]. This distinction is also clearly reflected in regulatory science. According to FDA standards, in vitro diagnostic devices (IVDs) intended for screening must meet stringent requirements: (1) high PPV in low-prevalence settings, (2) analysis of overdiagnosis/overtreatment risks due to false positives, (3) statistical validation based on prospective multicenter clinical trials, and (4) *demonstrate clinical benefit compared with or in combination with existing methods*. Furthermore, IVDs for screening must demonstrate high reproducibility, logistics suitable for large populations, cost-effectiveness, and integration with follow-up diagnostic pathways to gain market approval.

Despite these high entry barriers, liquid biopsy-based cancer screening methods are being actively developed worldwide as promising strategies to complement or replace conventional imaging and pathology tests. However, there remains a lack of standardized "clinical-grade" assays, and liquid biopsy technologies with sufficient sensitivity and specificity for early detec-

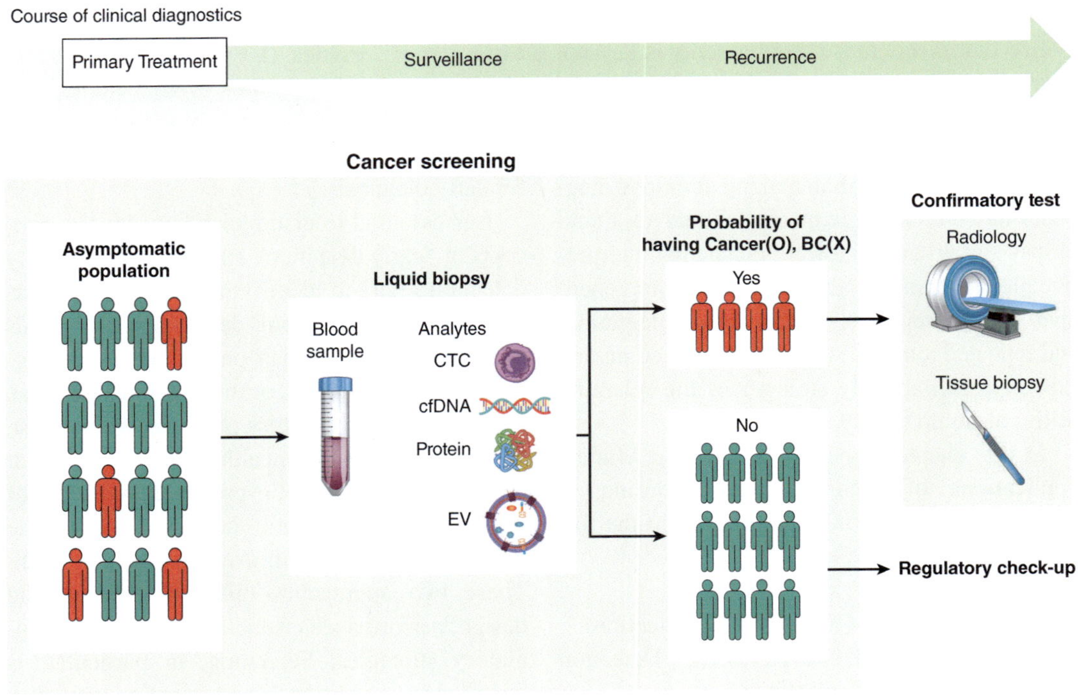

Fig. 5.2 Liquid biopsy–based assessment of cancer probability in screening

tion of solid tumors continue to represent an unmet medical need.

Liquid biopsy technologies for early cancer detection must address two key challenges: false negatives and false positives. False negatives in early-stage cancer can lead to missed diagnoses and delayed treatment, while false positives may result in unnecessary confirmatory tests, invasive procedures, and psychological distress for patients. Therefore, for the specific application of screening, it is essential to establish clinical utility, including PPV and NPV, in addition to sensitivity and specificity. PPV is directly related to the burden of false positives, while NPV ensures the reliability of negative results; both are considered key performance indicators in cancer screening.

Demonstrating such performance requires large-scale prospective clinical studies in the general population. In real-world screening settings, it is necessary to validate biomarker expression patterns in asymptomatic individuals, and analytical technologies capable of identifying tumor molecular heterogeneity and tissue of origin (TOO) are essential to ensure diagnostic utility. These are also core technical requirements in the development of multi-cancer early detection (MCED) tests.

Potential biomarkers for early diagnosis under investigation include CTCs, ctDNA, cfDNA, cfDNA methylation patterns, cfDNA fragmentation patterns, and exosomal RNA/miRNA, each with distinct technical advantages and limitations. For example, ctDNA analysis based on cfDNA enables highly sensitive detection of specific gene mutations; however, in early-stage cancer, the variant allele frequency (VAF) is extremely low, limiting sensitivity and resulting in potential detection failures. In contrast, cfDNA methylation pattern analysis offers tissue specificity, which is advantageous for tissue of origin (TOO) identification, but the process is complex and costly. CTCs allow for proteomic and transcriptomic analysis at the single-cell level, but their low abundance in blood leads to very low detection rates, and standardization of isolation techniques remains insufficient. Extracellular vesicles (EVs) are notable for their stability and suitability for multi-omics analysis; however, because the majority of circulating EVs originate from normal cells, ensuring tumor specificity remains a major challenge, in addition to the technical hurdles of selective isolation. Therefore, at present, an integrated approach utilizing multiple analytes according to the analytical purpose and clinical scenario is considered a more practical strategy. This section aims to summarize recent clinical research findings focusing on representative platforms for ctDNA and cfDNA methylation pattern analysis—namely, CancerSeek, cfMeDIP-seq, DELFI, and Epi proColon—and the EV-based platform ExoDx Prostate.

First, the blood-based CancerSeek test [7], which utilizes multiple markers including ctDNA present in cell-free DNA and circulating proteins, has been reported. CancerSeek is a multi-marker assay that integrates ctDNA mutation analysis with the detection of eight circulating proteins, representing one of the first large-scale clinical attempts to combine cfDNA and protein biomarkers for early cancer detection. Specifically, it analyzes mutations in 16 driver genes in ctDNA and simultaneously evaluates eight circulating proteins, including CA-125, CEA, CA19-9, and prolactin. The resulting data are processed using machine learning algorithms to predict both the presence of cancer and the likely tissue of origin. In the initial report, validation was conducted in 1005 patients with nonmetastatic solid tumors and 812 healthy controls. Across eight major cancer types (ovary, liver, stomach, pancreas, esophagus, colon, lung, and breast), the test achieved an average sensitivity of 70% and specificity of 99%. However, there were marked differences by cancer stage: sensitivity was only 43% for stage I cancers, but increased to 78% for stage III and 93% for stage IV. Thus, a structural limitation of significantly reduced sensitivity in early-stage disease was evident. This trend was also observed in the large-scale prospective DETECT-A trial (NCT04213326). In this study, 10,006 asymptomatic adults participated, and overall specificity remained high at 98.9%, but sensitivity was only 27.1% [13]. Of the 26 cancer cases detected, only 5 (19%) were stage I and 3 (12%) were stage II, whereas 8 (31%) were stage III and 9 (35%) were stage IV, indicating that the majority were advanced cancers. In other words, approximately 65% of patients detected by CancerSeek were already at stage III or higher, highlighting the limitations of this test as a screening tool for early cancer detection. Moreover, CancerSeek was restricted to eight predefined cancer types and did not include some common malignancies such as prostate and brain cancers, limiting its generalizability. Additionally, CancerSeek faced inherent limitations in localizing the tumor of origin using ctDNA mutations alone. In the DETECT-A study, participants with positive blood test results required PET-CT (positron emission tomography-computed tomography) to confirm the final tumor location, resulting in additional procedural and financial burdens within the diagnostic workflow [13]. Nevertheless, the CancerSeek study holds historical significance as the first to demonstrate the feasibility of a multi-marker, liquid biopsy-based early detection strategy at a clinical scale. Notably, it was the first clinical validation of a multi-omics approach integrating cfDNA and protein markers, moving beyond the limitations of single-marker strategies and laying the conceptual foundation for next-generation platforms such as cfMeDIP-seq, DELFI, and Galleri. In summary, despite clear limitations in sensitivity and tissue localization, CancerSeek established the groundwork for liquid biopsy-based early cancer detection. It is regarded as a pioneering effort that expanded the paradigm of early diagnosis research to a new axis of "multi-marker-based and machine learning-integrated" approaches.

The lessons learned from CancerSeek subsequently led to the development of next-generation early cancer detection platforms. A representative example is CancerGuard. CancerGuard is a multi-cancer early detection (MCED) test under development by Exact Sciences, which builds upon the design of CancerSeek while evolving to integrate three tiers of biomarkers. Specifically, by introducing the MP-R (mutation, protein, methylation—risk integration) model that simultaneously analyzes genetic mutations, DNA methylation patterns, and circulating proteins,

CancerGuard addresses the limitations of single-marker approaches.

According to the ASCEND-2 Study (NCT04213326) reported at AACR 2024, CancerGuard demonstrated a clinical sensitivity of 50.9% across 21 cancer types. For stage I cancers, it showed approximately a 28% improvement in sensitivity compared to previous approaches, and the combined sensitivity for stage I/II cancers also improved by more than 12%. Additionally, for six cancer types with low 5-year survival rates, a clinical sensitivity of 63.7% was reported. These results indicate a substantial improvement in early cancer detection performance, suggesting meaningful clinical progress, particularly in screening settings for low-prevalence populations. Notably, despite improved sensitivity, specificity remained comparable to CancerSeek, suggesting that diagnostic performance was enhanced without a concomitant rise in false positives.

Furthermore, CancerGuard not only detects the presence of cancer but also enhances the accuracy of identifying the tissue of origin (TOO). The machine learning-based interpretive algorithm integrates cfDNA methylation signals and protein expression patterns to predict TOO, with preliminary clinical studies reporting a prediction accuracy exceeding 88%, although further validation in independent, peer-reviewed cohorts is needed to confirm these results. Simulation models projected that incorporating CancerGuard into standard screening could reduce cancer-related mortality by ~17% and stage IV incidence by ~42% over 10 years, although these findings remain model-based estimates rather than clinical trial outcomes.

Such performance improvements are understood as strategies to overcome the structural limitations revealed by CancerSeek. That is, while detection of early-stage cancer was limited when relying solely on ctDNA fragments, CancerGuard strengthened its capability to integratively capture even ultralow-abundance signals by combining multilayered biomarkers. In addition, by pre-designing the imaging resolution pathway, it was reported to have the potential to reduce unnecessary diagnostic procedures by about 30% following a positive blood test.

Ultimately, CancerGuard can be seen as an attempt that addresses the limitations of CancerSeek and achieves clinical advancement, representing the evolution toward a new framework of multi-biomarker, multi-omics, and AI-based analysis. This marks an important milestone, demonstrating that liquid biopsy-based early detection technologies are moving beyond the stage of mere possibility toward establishing clinical reliability and improving patient outcomes.

As illustrated by the above case, the most significant limitation of ctDNA-based blood tests for solid tumors is the low sensitivity in early-stage disease. This is fundamentally due to the extremely low concentration of tumor-derived DNA (fragmented ctDNA) in the blood. In early-stage tumors, the variant allele frequency (VAF) often falls below 0.1%, while cfDNA released from normal blood cells is present at relatively high concentrations, increasing the background noise in analysis. As a result, ultralow-abundance ctDNA signals are easily diluted and missed, directly leading to reduced diagnostic sensitivity. To overcome this, strategies such as expanding the target mutation panel or increasing the input amount of cfDNA to improve the signal-to-noise ratio are being explored.

Additionally, CHIP (clonal hematopoiesis of indeterminate potential) is also recognized as a significant confounding factor. CHIP refers to age-related somatic mutations in the hematopoietic stem cell compartment, which can introduce non-cancer-related mutations such as TP53, DNMT3A, and TET2 into cfDNA, potentially causing false positives. In the DETECT-A study, among 490 individuals initially testing positive, 214 were ultimately attributed to CHIP-related variants and excluded; after this correction, the final specificity remained high at 98.9%. In other words, CHIP is a biological confounding factor that must be carefully managed to minimize false positives in ctDNA-based early detection approaches [11, 12].

To address these limitations, recent attention has focused on technologies based on cfDNA methylation pattern analysis. A representative method, cfMeDIP-seq (cell-free methylated DNA immunoprecipitation sequencing), captures tissue-specific epigenetic alterations, enabling not only the detection of cancer presence but also the simultaneous prediction of the tissue of origin (TOO). Preliminary clinical trials have demonstrated its applicability across various solid tumors, including lung, liver, breast, pancreatic, and colorectal cancers. In early-stage (stage I–II) lung cancer patients, preliminary pilot studies reported sensitivity exceeding 80% and specificity above 95%, although these findings require further validation in larger prospective cohorts [14]. This is attributed to the biological characteristic that DNA methylation reflects both tumor and tissue specificity.

Notably, in 2024, Guardant SHIELD obtained FDA premarket approval (PMA) as the first blood-based colorectal cancer (CRC) screening test, marking a pivotal milestone in the clinical adoption of liquid biopsy for population-level cancer screening. The pivotal ECLIPSE study (NCT 04136002), a prospective multicenter clinical trial involving over 20,000 participants, reported an overall CRC sensitivity of 83%, stage I sensitivity of 65%, and specificity of 90% [15]. These results are significant in that, compared to colonoscopy or fecal immunochemical test (FIT), the test is less invasive, has higher compliance, and offers clinically acceptable accuracy. SHIELD has thus demonstrated its potential to fill the clinical gap between existing imaging and stool-based tests.

In the same indication, Freenome's PREEMPT CRC trial (NCT04369053) applied a multi-omics approach integrating cfDNA methylation, protein, and fragmentomics, reporting a CRC sensitivity of 79.2% and specificity of 91.5% [16]. This study suggested that algorithm-based data integration and multi-marker fusion can further optimize screening performance.

Another representative example of a methylation-based approach is Epi proColon. This test qualitatively assesses promoter methylation of the SEPTIN 9 gene and was developed as the first blood-based screening test for colorectal cancer (CRC) in average-risk individuals aged 50 and older. The clinical efficacy of Epi proColon has been evaluated in three major clinical trials.

In the first large-scale clinical trial, 1544 asymptomatic average-risk individuals were enrolled, with colonoscopy as the gold standard. The results showed a sensitivity of 68.2% and specificity of 80.0%. Notably, the positive predictive value (PPV) of 2.4% and the negative predictive value (NPV) of 99.7% reflect the actual screening performance in an asymptomatic population. The second trial directly compared Epi proColon with the fecal immunochemical test (FIT). Among 290 participants, Epi proColon demonstrated a sensitivity of 72.2% and specificity of 80.8%, while FIT showed a sensitivity of 68.0% and specificity of 97.4%. Thus, while Epi proColon improved sensitivity for early-stage CRC detection, its lower specificity and PPV compared to FIT were primarily attributable to an increased false-positive rate. The third trial assessed actual patient compliance, with 202 out of 203 recommended individuals undergoing the test, resulting in a very high compliance rate of 99.5%. This highlights the advantages of blood-based approaches in terms of patient convenience and compliance compared to colonoscopy or stool tests. However, due to its relatively low PPV and limited sensitivity for early-stage cancer, Epi proColon has not yet been included in the US USPSTF guidelines and is used only in a limited capacity in parts of Europe and China. In summary, while Epi proColon opened the door to commercialized blood-based early CRC testing, its performance limitations have prompted a transition to next-generation technologies. It holds historical significance in that it provided clinical lessons that highlighted the necessity of early cancer detection.

CancerSeek is regarded as a pivotal attempt that marked a major turning point in liquid biopsy-based early cancer detection research. While single-cancer, single-marker approaches such as the Epi proColon test using SEPT9 methylation have already been commercialized, these were limited to specific cancer types (e.g., colorectal cancer). In contrast, CancerSeek was designed to simultaneously detect eight major solid tumors by combining ctDNA mutation analysis with eight circulating proteins and, further, to predict the tissue of origin. As the first large-scale clinical validation of a multi-marker, multi-cancer approach, CancerSeek is regarded as a pioneering effort that established the conceptual foundation for today's multi-cancer early detection (MCED) research.

Subsequent studies, particularly those led by GRAIL, have focused on improving tissue specificity by profiling cfDNA methylation patterns, thereby moving beyond mutation-only detection. Notable examples include the CCGA study (Circulating Cell-free Genome Atlas, NCT02889978) and the STRIVE study (NCT03085888). The CCGA study is an observational cohort involving over 15,000 participants, conducting detailed analyses of cfDNA methylation signals across various cancer types. The STRIVE study is a prospective, breast cancer-focused study involving over 100,000 women, simultaneously validating cancer signal detection and tissue of origin (TOO) prediction.

A combined analysis of these two studies demonstrated an overall sensitivity of 43.9% at a specificity of 99.3% across more than 50 cancer types, and a sensitivity of 67.3% for 12 predefined major cancers. By stage, the sensitivity was 39% for Stage I, 69% for Stage II, 83% for Stage III, and 92% for Stage IV, indicating higher detection rates in advanced cancers but still limited sensitivity in early stages. Importantly, the combined CCGA and STRIVE analyses achieved approximately 93% accuracy in tissue-of-origin prediction, providing robust evidence of the clinical potential of cfDNA methylation profiling. This represents a significant advance over previous limitations, such as CancerSeek's reliance on adjunct imaging modalities like PET-CT for localization, and provides the first large-scale clinical evidence—through the CCGA and STRIVE studies—that cfDNA methylation profiling can both detect cancer and accurately predict the tissue of origin.

GRAIL's Galleri test is a representative MCED platform that utilizes methylation pattern analysis of cfDNA to simultaneously determine the presence of cancer and its tissue of origin (TOO). This approach is distinguished from conventional ctDNA mutation analysis by not being limited to mutation detection, but by leveraging machine learning algorithms to interpret epigenetic signatures, thereby identifying tissue specificity for each cancer type. In fact, methylation data from large-scale cohorts such as CCGA and STRIVE formed the basis for the development of the Galleri algorithm, enabling MCED platforms to include tissue of origin prediction accuracy as a key performance metric, in addition to sensitivity and specificity. Currently, MCED development is transitioning from the stage of large-scale cohort-based methylation signature discovery to the phase of multicenter, prospective RCT-based clinical utility validation.

A representative example is the PATHFINDER study (NCT04241796). This multicenter, prospective evaluation enrolled 6621 participants who underwent the Galleri test, with 92 actual cancer cases diagnosed. Notably, 48% of these were detected at early stages (Stage I–II). Compared to the stage distribution under standard of care (SOC), Galleri demonstrated a clear stage shift, with a higher proportion of cancers diagnosed at Stage I–II compared to standard of care. While this stage shift indicates earlier detection, long-term survival benefit remains to be confirmed through randomized trials such as PATHFINDER-2. Cancer site prediction accuracy was 88%, and the median time to diagnostic resolution was approximately 79 days, highlighting both accuracy and workflow efficiency. Thus, Galleri demonstrated improved early detection rates and diagnostic efficiency. This study provides critical evidence for how MCED can be integrated into real-world clinical workflows and is regarded as the first case to quantitatively validate the clinical utility of liquid biopsy-based early cancer detection strategies.

The subsequent PATHFINDER-2 study (NCT05155605) was designed as a randomized clinical trial (RCT) to evaluate whether the Galleri-based MCED strategy could improve early cancer detection rates and survival outcomes in real-world clinical settings. According to results published in 2025, PATHFINDER-2 was a prospective, multicenter interventional study that assessed the safety and efficacy of Galleri in approximately 35,000 individuals aged 50 and older who were eligible for cancer screening, based on the number and types of diagnostic evaluations performed in participants with detected cancer signals. In the PATHFINDER study, Galleri demonstrated a positive predictive value (PPV) of 43%—that is, the probability that a positive result was confirmed as cancer—a specificity of 99.5%, and a cancer signal origin (CSO) accuracy of 88%. Data from evaluable PATHFINDER-2 participants after 12 months of follow-up showed a significantly higher PPV than observed in the original PATHFINDER study. CSO accuracy and specificity were consistent with those previously reported, and no serious safety issues were identified. The fact that the direct impact of MCED platforms, including Galleri, on actual patient care pathways is now being demonstrated at the level of large-scale, multicenter RCTs is highly significant. Thus, the Galleri and PATHFINDER studies indicate that liquid biopsy-based early cancer detection is moving beyond mere technical feasibility to a stage where it can drive changes in clinical workflows and contribute to improved patient outcomes. This represents a transition of MCED from a "discovery" tool to a "clinical tool"[8, 17].

DELFI (DNA Evaluation of Fragments for Early Interception) [18] is a novel early cancer detection strategy that utilizes the fragmentation patterns of cfDNA (fragmentomics). Instead of directly detecting genetic mutations, this technology analyzes DNA fragment length distributions and nucleosome positioning patterns to capture cancer-specific signals. The underlying concept is that cfDNA released from normal cells exhibits a relatively uniform distribution centered around 160–180 bp due to regular nucleosome organization, whereas cfDNA derived from tumor cells forms irregular and asymmetric fragment length patterns due to abnormal regulation of apoptosis and chromatin instability. These differences are leveraged through statistical modeling and machine learning algorithms to effectively distinguish cancer patients from healthy individuals. In initial validation studies, DELFI achieved 98% specificity with sensitivities ranging from 57 to 99% depending on cancer type, though further prospective validation is required to confirm these results. Furthermore, by applying machine learning algorithms to cfDNA fragment patterns, the tissue of origin (TOO) of tumors was successfully predicted in approximately 75% of patients. This represents an innovative approach that addresses the limitations of mutation-based ctDNA analysis and demonstrates the potential to improve sensitivity, particularly in cancers with low mutational burden or at early stages. Currently, multiple prospective clinical studies of the DELFI platform are underway, primarily focused on lung cancer. Notable examples include the DNA Evaluation of Fragments for Early Interception—Lung Cancer Training Study (NCT04825834) and the CASCADE-LUNG trial (NCT05306288), which is being conducted simultaneously at multiple sites in the USA and Europe. These studies aim to evaluate the clinical utility of DELFI-based screening in asymptomatic high-risk populations and are designed to compare its performance with existing low-dose CT (LDCT) and assess their potential complementarity. Notably, a 2024 report demonstrated that integrating DELFI fragmentomics with protein markers could further enhance early lung cancer detection performance. Compared to cfDNA fragmentomics analysis alone, both sensitivity and tumor localization accuracy were significantly improved, suggesting that a multimodal approach is key to optimizing early detection performance. These findings are being further validated in large-scale prospective studies such as the CASCADE-LUNG trial, strongly supporting the potential of the DELFI platform to evolve from a research tool into a clinically applicable early cancer screening technology. On the conceptual foundation established by CancerSeek–CancerGuard, next-generation platforms such as cfDNA methylation pattern analysis (cfMeDIP-seq, Galleri) and cfDNA fragmentomics (DELFI) have rapidly emerged, advancing ctDNA-based early cancer screening beyond the realm of mere feasibility studies.

These technologies are now entering the stage of clinical implementation, supported by regulatory approvals (e.g., FDA-approved Guardant SHIELD, CE-IVD certified platforms) and large-scale prospective clinical trials (CCGA, PATHFINDER, NHS-Galleri, CASCADE-LUNG). This demonstrates that liquid biopsy can introduce a new paradigm of simultaneous multi-cancer early detection (MCED)—a capability not offered by conventional imaging or tissue biopsy—into the field of public health. Ultimately, ctDNA-based MCED holds the potential not only to benefit individual patients but also to fundamentally transform the public health framework for cancer surveillance and screening. With accumulating evidence for earlier detection (stage shift), earlier therapeutic intervention, improved survival rates, and even changes in national-level healthcare resource allocation and cost-effectiveness, ctDNA-based early diagnosis research is expected to become a central pillar of future precision medicine and preventive oncology.

In addition, early diagnostic technologies utilizing tumor-derived extracellular vesicles (tEVs) are gaining increasing attention. EVs are vesicles secreted from endosomal or plasma membrane origins and are stably present in various body fluids, including the blood. Notably, EVs function as sophisticated information carriers that selectively reflect the molecular characteristics of their cells of origin, rather than being mere cellular debris. Tumor-derived EVs carry cancer-specific biomolecules such as miRNA, lncRNA, DNA fragments, and tumor-specific proteins, enabling the simultaneous achievement of tissue specificity and cancer specificity through their analysis. Due to their lipid bilayer structure, EVs protect their internal nucleic acids and proteins from external enzymes and nucleases, resulting in high stability in the bloodstream. This confers advantages over cfDNA or circulating RNA in terms of long-term storage and repeated sample collection, making EVs well-suited for actual clinical workflows. Furthermore, EVs can provide integrated multi-omics information—including nucleic acids, proteins, lipids, and metabolites—offering a multicomponent diagnostic window that can overcome the limitations of single-marker approaches, especially in the context of early-stage cancers where biomarkers are present at extremely low levels. A representative commercial example is ExoDx Prostate (IntelliScore, EPI). This test targets male patients with PSA levels in the 2–10 ng/mL "gray zone," analyzing the combined expression of three exosomal RNAs (PCA3, ERG, SPDEF) extracted from urine-derived EVs. The test has been shown to effectively stratify patients with high-risk prostate cancer (Gleason score $\geq$ 7) into high- and low-risk groups. ExoDx Prostate is clinically significant not as a screening tool for asymptomatic adults, but as a means to reduce unnecessary tissue biopsies and more accurately identify high-risk patients in populations where PSA testing alone yields diagnostic uncertainty. In several prospective clinical studies, this test has been reported to reduce unnecessary biopsies by approximately 27%. Based on this evidence, it has been included in the NCCN Prostate Cancer Early Detection v1.2023 guidelines and has received FDA Breakthrough Device designation. Beyond this, active research is underway on EV-based early diagnosis across various cancer types. The most well-known example of EV-based early cancer detection is the identification of Glypican-1 (GPC1)-expressing EVs in the blood of pancreatic cancer patients [19]. This study demonstrated that GPC1+ EVs in the blood can be detected with high sensitivity and specificity even in early-stage pancreatic cancer. However, subsequent studies reported inconsistent reproducibility, and thus, the role of GPC1+ EVs remains debated. Notably, this approach overcame the limitations of conventional serum CA19–9 testing, clearly distinguishing pancreatic cancer patients from those with chronic pancreatitis, and showed that postoperative changes in EV levels correlated with prognosis. This indicates that EV represents the first clinical evidence demonstrating that protein markers can surpass conventional serum protein-based diagnostic methods and is regarded as a landmark achievement in EV-based early cancer detection research. Subsequent studies have further expanded the potential of EVs for early cancer diagnosis. Large-scale EV proteomic analyses have compared the protein composition of blood EVs from patients with various cancer types, revealing that EV surface protein patterns exhibit cancer type-specific signatures [20]. These findings suggest that EV protein profiles may be useful for predicting the tissue of origin (TOO) of cancers. A recent large-scale study analyzed over 400 EV samples worldwide through a multicenter network. This research demonstrated that EV proteins can reflect not only early cancer detection but also organotropic metastasis, thereby further expanding the clinical applicability of EV analysis. However, controversy remains regarding the presence of nucleic acids (cargo nucleic acids) within EVs. For example, one study separated EVs from non-vesicular extracellular particles (NVEPs) and analyzed the molecular content of the cargo, finding that a significant portion of miRNA and cfDNA signals previously attributed to EVs actually originated from non-vesicular extracellular particles (e.g., RNP complexes) [21]. This study concluded that small EVs (exosomes) may not stably encapsulate nucleic acids, raising concerns about the interpretation of EV-based nucleic acid biomarkers. However, this remains controversial, as other reports have provided evidence for nucleic acid cargo within EVs. Thus, while EV research offers attractive possibilities for the discovery of tumor-specific protein and RNA markers, it is fundamentally limited by the fact that cargo composition and interpretation can vary greatly depending on the isolation method used. To date, a variety of EV isolation techniques—including ultracentrifugation, size-exclusion chromatography, immunoaffinity capture, and microfluidics—have been employed, often in multi-modal approaches. However, there is still no internationally agreed-upon standardized protocol, with only recommendations currently available. Such technical heterogeneity makes it difficult to compare results across studies and represents the greatest barrier to ensuring reproducibility in clinical applications. Ultimately, for EV-based early cancer diagnostic platforms to achieve clinical reliability, it is essential to establish standardized definitions and protocols for EV isolation and purification, reach consensus on the presence of EV cargo, and develop strategies to eliminate non-EV contaminant signals. In summary, EV-based early cancer diagnostic technologies can overcome the limitations of conventional ctDNA-only approaches through three key features: excellent stability, provision of multilayered molecular information, and the potential for organ and cancer type specificity. Some studies have shown that integrating cfDNA-based analysis with EV protein analysis significantly improves screening accuracy. These results suggest that EVs can function not only as standalone analytes but also as core components of multi-omics-based integrated early diagnostic platforms. Currently, commercialization has been achieved only for a limited number of cancer types, such as ExoDx Prostate. However, with large-scale prospective clinical trials and international standardization efforts, EVs have great potential to become next-generation key analytes in the field of cancer screening and early detection. In addition to the ctDNA- and EV-based early diagnostic and screening approaches discussed above, readers may wonder why circulating tumor cell (CTC)-based diagnostic methods have not been introduced. Theoretically, CTCs provide the most definitive "tumor-origin signal" as they offer direct cellular-level information. However, in early-stage cancers, the number of CTCs in the blood is extremely low (typically fewer than 1–10 per 10^6–10^7 leukocytes), making stable and reliable detection technically challenging. Therefore, CTCs are currently considered more suitable for prognosis prediction and treatment response monitoring in early cancer patients, rather than for screening purposes. Indeed, studies have reported that the presence of CTCs in preoperative blood samples from early breast cancer patients is significantly associated with recurrence-free survival, and some clinical studies have shown that CTC detection can serve as a prognostic factor for the early identification of patients at high risk of metastasis [22–24]. This will be discussed in detail in the following section.

In addition to cfDNA, EVs, and CTCs, tumor-educated platelets (TEPs) have also been investigated as analytes for early diagnosis. Platelets undergo selective alterations in their RNA profiles in response to EVs, cytokines, and growth factors released from tumor cells, thereby reflecting cancer-specific transcriptomic signals. Initial reports suggested that platelet RNA-seq analysis could distinguish cancer patients from controls with over 96% accuracy, although large-scale validation and reproducibility across independent cohorts remain lacking [25]. These findings suggest that TEPs could serve as a novel candidate for blood-based MCED, and the establishment of preprocessing and standardization technologies remains a challenge.

Furthermore, individual circulating microRNAs (miRNAs), circulating proteins, or their combinations (signatures) are also being studied as early diagnostic biomarkers. In various cancer types, certain molecules have been consistently reported to be overexpressed in the plasma of early-stage cancer patients, and multiple candidate panels have demonstrated the potential for early cancer detection. However, the analysis of these circulating molecules has not yet reached clinical standardization due to issues such as a lack of reproducibility across platforms and variability depending on preprocessing conditions.

In summary, while ctDNA and EVs currently form the core of early detection research, other analytes such as CTCs, TEPs, miRNAs, and proteins are also being studied in parallel, each with their own unique advantages. Although these analytes face significant limitations for use as standalone screening tests, they may serve as complementary components in multi-omics and multi-analyte integrated strategies, potentially improving both the sensitivity and specificity of early cancer screening.

In conclusion, it is important to recognize that liquid biopsy-based strategies for early detection and screening of solid tumors must go beyond demonstrating technical performance and provide evidence of actual clinical benefit to patients. In addition to improvements in analytical sensitivity and clinical performance resulting from technological advances, a multidimensional assessment of clinical utility—including impact on clinical decision-making, patient outcome improvement, and cost-benefit analysis—is essential.

From this perspective, leading platforms such as GRAIL's Galleri test have attracted significant global attention. As previously described, the Galleri test employs cfDNA methylation patterns to detect more than 50 types of solid tumors and predict the tissue of origin (TOO), presenting a multi-cancer early detection (MCED) strategy. This approach has been evaluated in clinical studies such as CCGA (NCT02889978) and PATHFINDER (NCT04241796), and in the UK, the NHS-Galleri Trial (NCT05611632) is being conducted as a large-scale randomized controlled clinical trial. Notably, the ongoing NHS-Galleri Trial is establishing itself as a key example for verifying whether liquid biopsy can contribute to earlier detection and improved survival in real patients, by comparing changes in stage distribution at diagnosis between the intervention and Standard of Care (SOC) groups through a "stage shift" analysis.

Ultimately, such large-scale multicenter clinical trials must provide concrete evidence of improved patient outcomes, beyond merely demonstrating technical performance, for early detection technologies to be adopted in clinical practice. To this end, long-term prospective studies in asymptomatic general populations are required, and clinical outcome measures such as overall survival, disease-free survival, and quality of life must be evaluated alongside diagnostic accuracy. At the same time, it is necessary to quantify the risks of overtreatment due to false positives and increased unnecessary procedures and to conduct cost-effectiveness analyses based on a balanced assessment of benefits and risks. Only by meeting these criteria can in vitro diagnostic devices (IVDs) intended for screening purposes satisfy regulatory requirements.

As a strategy to overcome these challenges, multi-analyte integration is being actively explored. For example, combining cfDNA methylation patterns with EV-derived RNA or protein markers can compensate for the limitations of individual analytes, thereby improving both sensitivity and tumor localization specificity. In addition, multi-omics-based approaches are advantageous for detecting subtle signals in early-stage cancers, and when combined with artificial intelligence (AI)-based interpretation algorithms, they enable the precise extraction of meaningful molecular patterns from large-scale datasets. This goes beyond simple biomarker assays, allowing for the development of precision diagnostic models based on high-dimensional data integration. Such technological advances are gradually making early diagnosis a reality, and ultimately, the final goal must be to improve patient survival through large-scale prospective clinical trials. In the future, a precision medicine approach that incorporates liquid biopsy into risk-stratified screening models—taking into account cancer incidence, treatment outcomes, and the feasibility of early intervention for each cancer type—will be required. At the same time, for the practical implementation of multi-analyte diagnostic platforms, standardization of pre-analytical variables, adoption of automated workflows, and ensuring multicenter reproducibility are essential. However, this approach does not provide a "universal benefit" through early detection of all cancer types. Some cancers have relatively favorable prognoses even when diagnosed at a later stage, while others have limited treatment outcomes even if detected early. Furthermore, early detection of biologically indolent tumors or subclinical cancers may not improve survival rates and could lead to unnecessary tests, procedures, and psychological burden. Therefore, the simplistic equation of "early detection = improved survival" must be reinterpreted, and qualitative indicators such as ease of therapeutic intervention after diagnosis, reduction of treatment burden, and improvement in patient quality of life should also be considered. Ultimately, early detection strategies based on liquid biopsy require comprehensive validation to determine whether they can provide real clinical benefit to patients, beyond technical feasibility. To this end, the use of multi-analyte approaches, standardized pre-analytical processes, AI-based interpretation, and long-term follow-up studies is essential. Only when all these elements are met can liquid biopsy truly cross the final threshold of clinical utility as a tool for early cancer screening.

5.2 Minimal Residual Disease (MRD) Detection and Recurrence Monitoring

Minimal residual disease (MRD) refers to a state in which a small number of cancer cells persist in the body after standard treatment, posing a continued risk of recurrence or metastasis even in patients who appear to be in complete remission [3]. Conventional diagnostic methods such as imaging or histopathological evaluation have difficulty detecting this minimal disease, so MRD is often described as the "shadow of invisible cancer" and has emerged as a key precision medicine indicator in posttreatment patient monitoring. Recent studies have introduced the concept of "molecular relapse," which assigns clinical significance to cases where liquid biopsy-based signals—such as ctDNA, CTCs, or EVs—become positive before radiological recurrence is confirmed [9, 10]. Molecular relapse has been reported to precede radiological recurrence by an average of 3–12 months (depending on cancer type) and is recognized as an important early signal that determines the timing of clinical intervention and patient prognosis (Fig. 5.3) [1, 9, 10].

Recently, the concept of MRD has evolved beyond simple recurrence prediction to become a key management element for tailoring treatment strategies and providing tangible clinical benefits to patients. For example, in patients confirmed to be MRD-negative after therapy, unnecessary adjuvant therapy can be avoided, thereby reducing toxic side effects and maintaining quality of life, and conversely, for patients in whom MRD is detected as positive, precise interventions such as considering intensified therapy or planning close follow-up can be implemented [26, 27]. Therefore, MRD assessment should go beyond a simple binary interpretation of "present/absent" to include dynamic indicators from serial measurements, such as the kinetics of ctDNA—clearance, reappearance, and changes in concentration (slope) [2, 28]. This quantitative and dynamic approach enables personalized risk stratification for each patient and serves as a basis for future decisions regarding treatment intensity (de-esca-

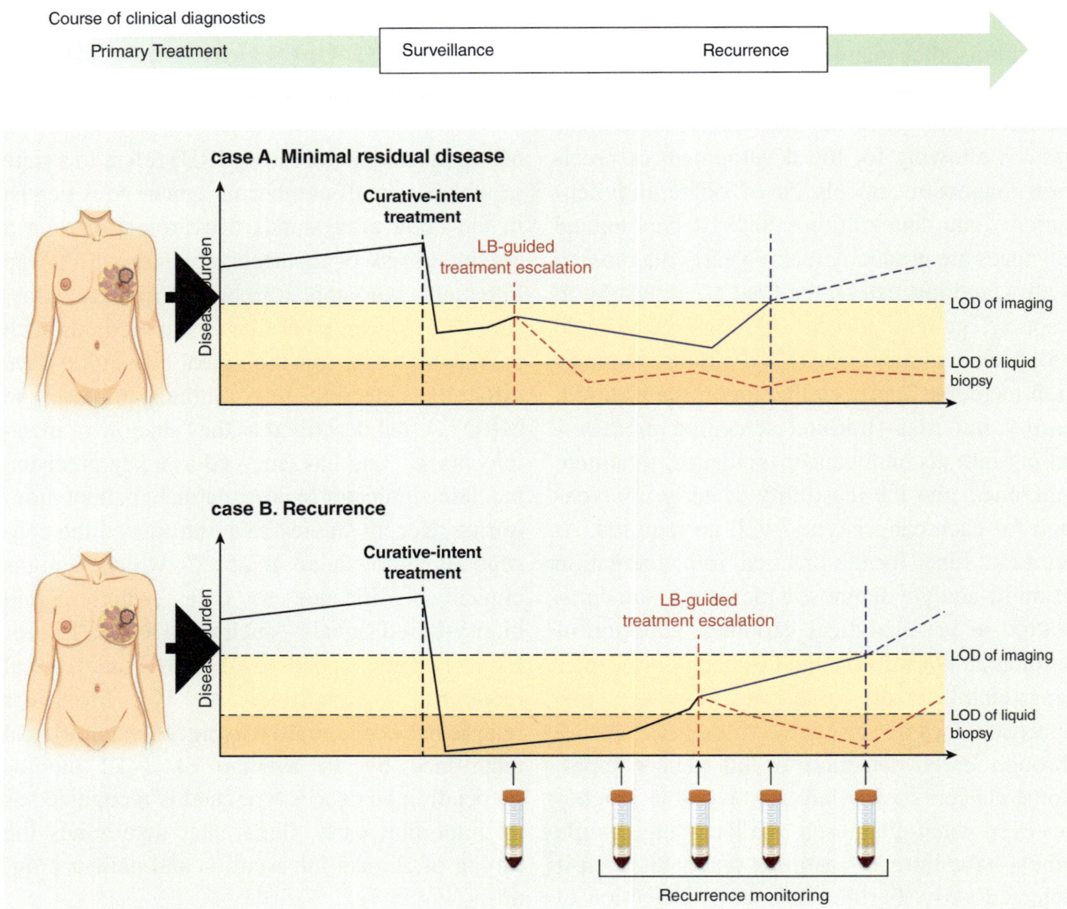

Fig. 5.3 Liquid biopsy for monitoring minimal residual disease and recurrence

lation vs. escalation). Among the various MRD assessment methods, liquid biopsy is currently the most prominent technology. Noninvasive, blood-based samples allow for repeated collection at multiple time points—immediately after surgery, during adjuvant chemotherapy, and at regular intervals after treatment—enabling the tracking of tumor kinetics. Liquid biopsy-based MRD detection can identify molecular signs of recurrence earlier than imaging modalities, with reports indicating detection on average 3–6 months and, in some studies, more than a year, before clinical relapse [9, 29]. Thus, MRD-based liquid biopsy provides temporal information that conventional static diagnostic methods cannot offer and is emerging as a technology that is transforming posttreatment patient management paradigms. Indeed, recent prospective clinical studies in colorectal and breast cancer have demonstrated that MRD-based decision-making can directly impact patient survival and treatment efficacy [27, 28]. The most representative analyte for MRD detection is ctDNA, which is currently the most actively developed and clinically applied field. ctDNA-based approaches are broadly divided into two categories. First, the "tumor-informed" approach, which identifies patient-specific tumor mutations in advance and tracks these mutations, allows for significantly increased sensitivity and specificity through customized probe design [10, 28]. Second, the "tumor-naïve" approach uses a fixed panel that includes mutations commonly found in specific cancer types, making it applicable even for patients from whom tumor tissue is difficult to obtain [30]. Numerous studies have demonstrated that ctDNA can be used for early MRD detection and recurrence risk prediction in colorectal cancer, bladder cancer, NSCLC, and others, thereby informing treatment strategies [1, 9, 29]. Representative commercial platforms include Natera's Signatera™, Inivata's RaDaR™, and Guardant's Reveal™ [10, 31]. Notably, Signatera™ has received breakthrough device designation from the FDA for MRD detection and has demonstrated a strong association between MRD positivity and recurrence risk in stage II colorectal cancer patients [26]. RaDaR™ is notable for its ability to detect ultralow frequency mutations by combining ultra-deep sequencing with error correction algorithms, while Guardant Reveal™ offers the advantage of MRD monitoring using only blood-based cfDNA panels without the need for tissue samples. CTCs are also being continuously evaluated as potential analytes for MRD detection. CTCs provide functional information beyond the DNA level, such as protein expression, EMT characteristics, and intercellular interactions, offering alternative value in cancer types where mutation-based approaches are challenging [32]. However, their extremely low concentration in the blood and the variability of results depending on the sensitivity and efficiency of detection technologies remain significant limitations. Recently, advances have been made in high-precision microfluidic separation technologies and antibody-based capture methods, and some studies suggest that phenotypic analysis of CTCs can be used to track clonal evolution in the MRD state or to predict the early emergence of therapy-resistant subclones. In particular, circulating tumor microemboli (CTM) are known to have higher metastatic potential than single CTCs, and their presence at the MRD stage has been linked to patient prognosis in recent research [33]. EVs are another promising analyte for MRD detection, offering advantages in terms of stability, inherent multiplexed biological information, and prolonged circulation in the bloodstream. Tumor-derived EVs contain selectively loaded miRNAs, methylated DNA, and tumor-associated proteins, and these signals can be utilized for early detection based on epigenetic signatures [20]. In particular, EVs remain stable in the bloodstream due to their lipid bilayer structure, and multi-omics analysis can be used to enhance both sensitivity and specificity. Early clinical studies suggest that combining EV-based MRD detection with ctDNA analysis may enhance sensitivity for recurrence prediction, although larger prospective validation is still needed [34]. However, the selective isolation of tumor-specific EVs remains a technical challenge, and research is ongoing into standardized preprocessing methods, surface marker-based purification technologies, and AI-driven pattern analysis. In summary, MRD-based liquid biopsy not only predicts recurrence but also directly influences the entire spectrum of clinical decision-making, including adjustment of treatment intensity, avoidance of unnecessary therapies, and improved precision in patient monitoring. For future advancement, it is essential to (1) continuously improve analytical sensitivity, (2) establish patient-specific MRD criteria, (3) conduct analyses linked to long-term clinical outcomes, (4) correct for biological variability arising from repeated measurements, and (5) perform multicenter, large-scale prospective cohort validation [3]. Ultimately, for MRD-based liquid biopsy to become a practical tool in precision medicine, it is necessary to integrate the strengths of each analyte and continuously accumulate scientific and clinical evidence to support patient-tailored monitoring strategies. This section provides a comprehensive review of the technical principles, representative platforms, clinical validation cases, recent prospective research trends, and future challenges for the implementation of these MRD-based analytes.

5.2.1 CTC (Circulating Tumor Cells)

CTC (circulating tumor cells)-based minimal residual disease (MRD) detection technologies depend critically on the precision of the entire process—preprocessing, separation, and detection—that efficiently enriches and preserves the minute quantities of cancer cells present in the bloodstream. This process goes beyond simple cell separation and requires multifaceted technical approaches that exploit the molecular and physical differences between cancer and non-cancer cells (such as surface proteins, size, density, deformability, and metabolic or secretory functions). To this end, the epithelial cell adhesion molecule (EpCAM) is known as the most widely used cell surface protein for CTC selection. EpCAM is overexpressed in many epithelial-derived cancers, making it useful for identifying CTCs; however, not all CTCs express EpCAM. In fact, during the epithelial-mesenchymal transition (EMT), cancer cells may reduce or lose EpCAM expression, which represents a significant limitation that can lead to the omission of CTCs during the separation process. For this reason, multi-marker approaches utilizing various epithelial cell surface antigens or tumor-specific antigens, in addition to EpCAM, have been attempted. However, CTCs are inherently highly heterogeneous in phenotype, and some CTCs may not express any of the conventionally defined surface markers. Therefore, single-marker-based positive selection methods not only fail to represent the entire CTC population by selecting only specific subtypes, but also carry the risk of false positives due to nonspecific binding of non-CTC cells. A strategy to overcome this limitation is negative selection. Negative selection methods use biomarkers not expressed by CTCs to remove nonspecific cells, allowing for the capture of a broader spectrum of CTCs. However, this approach also has drawbacks: compared to positive selection, the purity of the isolated CTC population is inevitably lower, and the absolute recovery rate and sensitivity for these rare cells in blood may be reduced. Recently, label-free approaches based on physical properties (e.g., size, density, deformability) have been developed. Although advanced separation techniques, including label-free isolation and microfluidics, are being developed, standardization and reproducibility for clinical application remain significant challenges. In fact, since the early 2020s, some size- and deformability-based technologies have entered the commercialization stage for clinical use, and devices such as Parsortix® offer workflows optimized for downstream analyses (genomic, proteomic, and single-cell omics) following antigen-independent cell collection. However, CTC isolation and enrichment methods based on physical properties such as size, density, and deformability have the limitation that the criteria for separation can vary depending on the technology used. These technical differences complicate the precise definition and comparative analysis of CTCs and may hinder interpretive consistency in clinical applications. CTC research is expanding beyond simple counting to include molecular characterization and functional analysis [35, 36]. Molecular analysis within single CTCs is a critical step following isolation, allowing for the identification of specific genetic mutations and expression patterns by combining immunostaining and fluorescence in situ hybridization (FISH). Furthermore, attempts are being made to obtain comprehensive genetic information from limited CTC samples through whole genome amplification (WGA) at the single-cell level. However, data obtained from single cells are subject to significant technical variability, which currently limits their application as a standardized (gold-standard) method in clinical practice. Additionally, approaches utilizing patient-derived xenograft (PDX) models are being explored to study the functional characteristics of CTCs and to assess drug responsiveness [35]. However, establishing PDX models requires several months, and successful engraftment and tumor formation necessitate a substantial number of homogeneous CTCs. Given the extremely low abundance of CTCs in blood, this presents a practical limitation. Therefore, to realize precision medicine based on liquid biopsy, it is essential to improve the sensitivity and accuracy of single-cell analysis technologies, develop efficient methods for establishing PDX models, and, most importantly, conduct large-scale prospective studies to demonstrate the clinical validity of these technologies. Despite these technological advances, clinical studies consistently demonstrate that CTCs can have real clinical value in MRD assessment. The concept that CTCs can be used to evaluate patient prognosis was first reported in 2004 [32]. A representative study in patients with metastatic breast cancer was the first to demonstrate a clear correlation between CTC count and survival. In this study, CTCs were measured in peripheral blood before treatment initiation in 177 patients with metastatic breast cancer using the CellSearch system. Patients with five or more CTCs per 7.5 mL of blood had significantly lower progression-free survival (PFS) and overall survival (OS) compared to those with fewer than five CTCs. Specifically, the median PFS and OS in the high CTC group (≥5 cells) were 2.7 months and 10.1 months, respectively, whereas in the low CTC group (<5 cells), the median PFS and OS were 7.0 months and 18.0 months, respectively. Multivariate analysis confirmed that the presence of CTCs was an independent prognostic factor and a sensitive biomarker capable of reflecting treatment response and disease progression at an early stage. This study is regarded as a landmark, demonstrating that CTCs are not merely byproducts of tumors but are biomarkers directly associated with cancer progression. Subsequent follow-up studies monitored CTC levels dynamically through repeated blood sampling during the course of treatment in the same patient cohort [37]. In 177 patients with metastatic breast cancer, CTCs were measured at regular intervals after the initiation of therapy, and it was confirmed that not only the baseline CTC count but also changes in CTC levels during treatment were closely associated with patient prognosis. The results showed that patients whose CTC counts remained at or above five or increased during treatment had significantly lower progression-free survival (PFS) and overall survival (OS). Specifically, in the group of patients with persistently high CTC levels, the median PFS was reported as 2.1 months and OS as 8.2 months. In contrast, in the group where CTC counts decreased during treatment, PFS was 7.0 months and OS was 21.3 months. These results demonstrate that CTCs are not limited to single-point detection but serve as dynamic biomarkers that reflect treatment response and disease progression in real time. In conclusion, CTC monitoring offers the potential for early assessment of treatment response and identification of patients with poor prognosis, enabling the development of personalized therapeutic strategies. This indicates that CTCs can function as quantitative indicators reflecting cancer progression, rather than merely being biological byproducts. Subsequent studies have shown that changes in CTC counts during treatment are directly linked to prognosis, further supporting the use of CTCs as dynamic biomarkers. Based on these findings, the CellSearch system has been recognized as a prognostic tool for not only metastatic breast cancer but also prostate and colorectal cancers, becoming the first liquid biopsy platform to receive FDA approval in the United States [38, 39].

In the mid-2000s, when the CELLSEARCH system began to be recognized as a prognostic factor in metastatic cancer, a new complementary approach was reported: the detection of cytokeratin-19 (CK-19) mRNA-positive CTCs in peripheral blood [22]. Unlike CELLSEARCH, this method does not directly isolate CTCs; instead, it separates PBMCs (peripheral blood mononuclear cells) from the blood, extracts RNA, and then detects the presence of CK-19 mRNA using real-time PCR.

This approach was applied to 167 patients with stage I–III early breast cancer, analyzing CK-19 mRNA-positive CTCs before the initiation of adjuvant chemotherapy. The study found that CK-19 mRNA-positive CTCs were detected in 47% of all patients, and these patients had significantly lower disease-free survival (DFS) and overall survival (OS) compared to those without CK-19 mRNA detection. Specifically, the 5-year DFS and OS rates for CK-19 mRNA-positive patients were 49% and 62%, respectively, whereas those for CK-19 mRNA-negative patients were 78% and 88%. Multivariate analysis also confirmed CK-19 mRNA positivity as an independent prognostic factor (HR = 2.08, $p = 0.001$). This study demonstrated that even in early breast cancer patients without metastasis, CTCs—particularly CK-19 mRNA-positive CTCs—are closely associated with recurrence and survival, highlighting the potential of noninvasive methods for evaluating MRD and prognosis.

In a subsequent study using the same system, it was confirmed that patients with detectable CK-19 mRNA-positive CTCs 2 years after completion of chemotherapy had a significantly higher risk of recurrence. Further research reported that detection of CTCs within 5 years after breast cancer diagnosis, especially in HER2-negative breast cancer patients, was associated with a markedly increased risk of recurrence [40]. In this study, among 353 hormone receptor-positive patients, the annual recurrence rate was 21.5% in CTC-positive patients, compared to only 2% in CTC-negative patients.

These studies have established CTCs as powerful biomarkers capable of predicting long-term prognosis not only in metastatic disease but also in early breast cancer patients. In particular, the CK-19 mRNA-based approach suggests the possibility of noninvasively estimating MRD and residual tumor cells. However, since this method does not isolate the cells themselves, further cellular-level analyses are not possible, limiting its utility for precision medicine applications that require direct cellular characterization.

In summary, CellSearch defines CTCs by combining EpCAM antibody-based positive selection with CK+/CD45− immunofluorescence staining and has received FDA approval for prognostic use in metastatic breast, prostate, and colorectal cancers. This landmark represents the first official clinical validation of CTCs, but also clearly revealed its limitations. The EpCAM-dependent isolation method fails to capture CTCs that have undergone EMT or possess atypical phenotypes, and in clinical research settings, issues of low sensitivity and limited reproducibility have been repeatedly raised [33].

To overcome these limitations, various next-generation CTC platforms are being developed. Parsortix® (ANGLE plc) utilizes microfluidic technology based on CTC size and deformability, enabling the capture of CTCs regardless of EpCAM expression. This is particularly advantageous for detecting EMT-CTCs or mesenchymal CTCs, thereby expanding the spectrum of CTCs captured compared to CellSearch. In 2022, it received FDA approval for CTC isolation in patients with metastatic breast cancer, making it the second platform to achieve regulatory success after CellSearch. ClearCell® FX (Biolidics) employs inertial microfluidics to continuously separate rare cells from blood samples. This technology boasts high purity and recovery rates, with particular strength in the immediate processing of fresh blood samples. The RareCyte® system combines slide-based high-resolution microscopic imaging with single-cell picking, enabling not only enumeration but also molecular analysis (DNA, RNA, protein) of individual CTCs. This addresses the major limitation of CellSearch, which lacked functional and molecular characterization capabilities. These next-generation platforms commonly overcome EpCAM dependency, capture a broader spectrum of rare CTCs, and extend capabilities from simple enumeration to molecular and functional analyses. However, they have not yet achieved widespread clinical adoption, with most remaining at the research-use-only (RUO) stage. Therefore, at present, CTC-based MRD detection is at a developmental stage where next-generation platforms such as Parsortix, ClearCell, and RareCyte complement the historical and clinical foundation provided by CellSearch with enhanced sensitivity, diversity, and molecular analysis capabilities. Moving forward, a key challenge in CTC research will be whether these technologies can surpass the limitations of CellSearch through large-scale prospective clinical trials and international standardization. Additionally, one study analyzed the correlation between CTC status, radiotherapy benefit, and survival in patients with early breast cancer [41]. In this study, CTCs were analyzed from blood samples collected prior to treatment initiation in patients who had undergone surgery for early-stage breast cancer, and the results were evaluated in relation to radiotherapy administration and long-term patient survival. Approximately 20% of the entire cohort were found to be CTC-positive before treatment, and these patients had a higher overall risk of recurrence and mortality compared to the CTC-negative group. Notably, in the CTC-positive group, radiotherapy significantly improved overall survival (OS). Specifically, CTC-positive patients who received radiotherapy had more than a 50% reduction in mortality risk compared to those who did not, with a significant difference also observed in 5-year follow-up survival rates. In contrast, among CTC-negative patients, there was no statistically significant difference in survival according to radiotherapy status. In other words, the clinical benefit of radiotherapy was clearly evident only in the high-risk group with detectable CTCs in the blood. These findings demonstrate that CTCs can function not only as prognostic biomarkers reflecting patient outcomes but also as predictive biomarkers for specific treatment efficacy. That is, CTC-positive patients are more likely to derive actual survival benefit from radiotherapy, while CTC-negative patients may avoid unnecessary treatment interventions, thereby preserving quality of life. In this context, CTC detection could serve as an important reference indicator for establishing personalized treatment strategies regarding radiotherapy decisions. This provides important clinical evidence suggesting that CTCs can directly contribute to clinical decision-making as a "stratification tool for treatment intensity adjustment." Furthermore, the GeparQuattro trial evaluated the prognostic value of CTCs before and after neoadjuvant chemotherapy (NAC) in patients with operable or locally advanced breast cancer [24]. In this study, blood samples were collected and CTCs analyzed from 213 patients both before treatment initiation and after completion of NAC. The results showed that patients with detectable CTCs prior to treatment exhibited significantly lower disease-free survival (DFS) and overall survival (OS). Notably, patients in whom CTCs persisted even after completion of neoadjuvant chemotherapy (NAC) had the poorest prognosis, which was closely associated with residual disease unresponsive to therapy. Specifically, patients who were CTC-positive before NAC had higher hazard ratios for both DFS and OS compared to CTC-negative patients, and those with persistent CTCs after NAC showed markedly increased rates of recurrence and mortality. In patient stratification based on changes in CTC status before and after NAC, those who converted to CTC-negative status demonstrated significantly better clinical outcomes than those who remained CTC-positive. This suggests that CTCs serve not only as a prognostic marker prior to treatment but also as a response marker reflecting NAC efficacy. This study demonstrated that CTC monitoring can play a crucial role in patient stratification and risk assessment during the formulation of treatment strategies. In particular, the persistence of CTCs in the bloodstream after NAC may serve as an early warning signal for residual disease and future recurrence risk, highlighting the need for intensified therapy or close surveillance. Therefore, the GeparQuattro trial is regarded as a study that established the clinical value of CTCs not merely as tumor byproducts, but as meaningful indicators of therapeutic response and prognostic prediction. Recent findings indicate that CTCs can exist not only as single cells but also in cluster forms (circulating tumor cell clusters or circulating tumor microemboli), and these CTC clusters have been reported to possess much higher metastatic potential and survival in the bloodstream than single CTCs [33]. CTC clusters are considered byproducts of collective cell migration during metastasis and, compared to single CTCs, exhibit enhanced survival and metastatic efficiency through cell–cell adhesion and interactions with tumor microenvironment-associated cells (e.g., fibroblasts, immune cells). CTC clusters display increased intravascular survival and metastatic capability, which are closely linked to cancer progression and prognosis. Notably, CTC clusters show resistance to apoptosis in the bloodstream, and epigenetic programs such as DNA methylation induce transcriptional profiles distinct from those of single CTCs, thereby enhancing stemness and metastatic capacity. Indeed, studies in animal models and patient-derived samples have shown that CTC clusters are 20–50 times more likely to initiate metastasis than single CTCs. These characteristics suggest that CTC clusters may have significant clinical implications as indicators of recurrence risk during the MRD (minimal residual disease) phase. In other words, the detection of CTC clusters in the blood after surgery or chemotherapy may signal not just the presence of residual cells, but the persistence of a tumor population with high metastatic potential. Therefore, detection of CTC clusters may serve as a stronger prognostic indicator in MRD assessment than enumeration of single CTCs. However, research on the biological characteristics and clinical significance of CTC clusters remains in its early stages, and clear criteria and functional roles need to be established. To date, the definition, detection criteria, and biological significance of CTC clusters vary across studies, and standardization is still lacking. The classification of "clusters" differs depending on size, cell number, and accompanying cell types, making cross-study comparisons challenging—a major limitation. Future research should employ single-cell transcriptomics and spatial multi-omics to elucidate the origin, functional heterogeneity, and direct association of CTC clusters with metastatic potential. In conclusion, CTC clusters are emerging not merely as aggregates of rare circulating cells but as key metastatic drivers and high-risk biomarkers for recurrence during the MRD phase and may become critical targets for early therapeutic intervention in the era of precision medicine.

The clinical utility of CTCs is now expanding beyond the context of MRD to serve as a predictive biomarker and decision-support tool for actual therapeutic decision-making. A representative example is the STIC CTC trial [42, 43]. This prospective, randomized clinical trial compared treatment selection strategies between endocrine therapy and chemotherapy in patients with hormone receptor-positive/HER2-negative metastatic breast cancer, based on CTC counts at the initiation of treatment. In the study, patients with ≥5 CTCs per 7.5 mL of blood were defined as having a poor prognosis, and the clinical utility of CTC-based treatment decisions was evaluated in patient groups with discordance between clinical criteria and CTC indicators (clinical–CTC discordance).

As a result, in patients with low CTC counts, an endocrine therapy-first strategy was proven to be safe and effective. Conversely, in cases of clinical–CTC discordance, patients with high CTC counts who received chemotherapy tended to have better progression-free survival (PFS) and overall survival (OS). This provides important evidence that CTC enumeration can function not only as a prognostic marker but also as a predictive and decision-support biomarker for actual therapeutic selection.

Subsequent studies have further reinforced this concept. With larger patient cohorts and long-term follow-up data, it has been reported that CTC enumeration and dynamic changes can stratify the benefit of chemotherapy. In particular, for patients with baseline CTCs ≥5, upfront chemotherapy may offer a long-term prognostic advantage over endocrine therapy alone. Conversely, in patients with low CTC concentrations, unnecessary chemotherapy can be avoided, and management with endocrine-based therapy alone is sufficient.

These findings demonstrate that CTCs are evolving beyond the traditional framework of a "prognostic marker" to serve as a "predictive and decision-support biomarker" that can directly guide therapeutic strategy selection. Therefore, CTCs are expanding their role from merely assessing MRD or predicting recurrence to supporting the full spectrum of clinical decision-making, including modulation of treatment intensity, therapeutic selection, and avoidance of unnecessary toxicity, as a next-generation precision medicine tool.

However, CTCs are rare events in the bloodstream, and their low analytical sensitivity and clinical specificity present clear limitations for clinical application. As mentioned earlier, there remains controversy as to whether all cells isolated and defined as positive in peripheral blood are truly cancer cells, and the extremely low detection frequency greatly increases analytical variability. Due to these characteristics, there is a high risk of detection failure in early-stage cancer or MRD settings, leading to ongoing criticism that CTCs are not suitable as surveillance markers in actual clinical practice. In addition, many CTC–MRD studies reported to date have been limited to relatively small cohorts and retrospective designs, highlighting the need for large-scale prospective clinical trials and long-term follow-up studies to ensure clinical reliability.

To overcome these limitations, recent efforts have focused on the development of automated platforms and the establishment of standardized analytical protocols. For example, next-generation microfluidics-based CTC isolation devices and automated enumeration systems that combine high-resolution imaging technologies with artificial intelligence (AI) algorithms are being developed to enhance reproducibility and consistency of interpretation. Furthermore, international consortia (e.g., IMI CANCER-ID, BloodPAC) are working to standardize pre-analytical conditions, marker selection, and reporting criteria for CTC analysis, and these consensus-building processes are providing a critical foundation for the clinical implementation of CTCs.

Moreover, CTC analysis is expanding beyond simple cell counting to a multi-omics approach encompassing genomics, transcriptomics, proteomics, and epigenomics. At the single-cell level, simultaneous analysis of mutations, expression patterns, transcriptome networks, and drug resistance-related pathways can provide functional and phenotypic information that conventional ctDNA-based approaches cannot offer. As such multidimensional data accumulate, CTCs have the potential to evolve beyond simple prognostic markers into concrete decision-support tools, such as predictive markers for treatment response, determining the need for radiotherapy, or assessing immunotherapy responsiveness. Ultimately, for CTC-based MRD detection technologies to become practical clinical tools, several conditions must be met: the development of ultra-precise isolation and detection platforms to enhance sensitivity; the establishment of international standardization and regulatory acceptance; large-scale prospective cohort validation; and the integration of multi-omics and AI-based precision analysis technologies. When these requirements are fulfilled, CTCs may be established not merely as "byproducts of cancer," but as next-generation dynamic biomarkers that contribute to the development of personalized treatment strategies and the realization of precision oncology.

5.2.2 Circulating Tumor DNA

ctDNA-based minimal residual disease (MRD) detection technologies derive their clinical value from the ability to detect minute quantities of tumor-derived DNA remaining in the body after treatment with high sensitivity and specificity. Beyond simply confirming the presence or absence of genetic mutations, it is essential to precisely identify tumor-specific signals present in extremely low abundance among the overwhelmingly large amounts of non-tumor cell-free DNA (cfDNA) in the blood. This requires not only highly advanced analytical technologies but also a deep understanding of tumor biology. ctDNA is primarily released through cell death processes, such as apoptosis or necrosis, but the release patterns vary significantly depending on the physiological and pathological characteristics of the tumor [2, 44]. Emerging evidence suggests that, in addition to passive release, active secretion mechanisms involving extracellular vesicles (EVs) may also contribute. In highly vascularized tumors with active angiogenesis or those infiltrating surrounding tissues, physical damage to the tumor microenvironment (TME), hypoxia, and immune cell-mediated cytolysis act in concert to accelerate ctDNA release. Such ctDNA can originate not only from the primary tumor but also from metastatic sites, and therapeutic interventions—such as chemotherapy, radiotherapy, or targeted therapy—can increase ctDNA release as tumor cells are destroyed. Consequently, ctDNA can serve as a dynamic biomarker reflecting a patient's treatment response [2, 44]. In practice, a rapid decrease in ctDNA concentration immediately after surgery or chemotherapy can serve as a sensitive indicator of treatment efficacy, whereas persistent detection of ctDNA after a certain period posttreatment strongly suggests the presence of residual disease or a high risk of recurrence [2, 9, 10]. Tumor-specific somatic mutations released into the bloodstream exist in the form of ctDNA and are theoretically considered noninvasive molecular markers with high tumor specificity. However, these signals generally exist at extremely low variant allele frequencies (VAF), necessitating the use of highly sensitive platforms for detection. Thus, ctDNA, while presenting both biological and analytical challenges, is emerging as the most promising candidate biomarker for MRD detection and early recurrence prediction. Even after complete surgical resection of the primary tumor, ctDNA can sometimes be detected in the patient's blood, which holds clinically significant implications extending beyond a mere residual posttreatment signal [2, 10]. This is interpreted as ctDNA being released from micrometastases undetectable by imaging or histological evaluation or from disseminated tumor cells (DTCs) that remain dormant in peripheral blood or distant organs. In other words, ctDNA reveals that radiological complete remission does not necessarily indicate eradication of disease at the molecular level [9, 10].

However, even in these circumstances, the precise biological mechanisms underlying ctDNA release have not been fully elucidated. The pattern of ctDNA release may vary depending on the anatomical location of metastases, the histological characteristics of the cells, and the viability of residual disseminated tumor cells (DTCs). For example, patients with metastases to the lung, peritoneum, or central nervous system often exhibit relatively low variant allele frequencies (VAFs), which is interpreted as the result of complex factors such as the rate of tumor cell death, vascular permeability at the metastatic site, the degree of immune cell attack, or metabolic stress within the tumor microenvironment, all of which influence the amount of ctDNA released [11, 45].

By definition, minimal residual disease (MRD) refers to a state in which the absolute number of tumor cells present in the body is extremely low, and accordingly, the concentration of ctDNA is also minuscule. In fact, from the MRD perspective, ctDNA often constitutes less than 0.01% of total cell-free DNA (cfDNA) [11]. This makes detection extremely challenging in early-stage cancer patients or in those with minimal residual disease following surgery or chemotherapy. For instance, prospective studies in breast and colorectal cancer have repeatedly shown that ctDNA can be detected on average 3 to 10 months before radiological recurrence, but these results were only possible with the application of ultrasensitive technologies [2, 9, 10].

Therefore, MRD monitoring requires the adoption of highly sensitive technologies such as ultra-deep sequencing, droplet digital PCR (ddPCR), and BEAMing [2]. These methods are designed to reliably detect trace amounts of tumor-specific mutations in individual patients, thereby lowering the detection limit and, when combined with longitudinal sampling strategies, enabling more precise assessment of MRD status. Large-scale prospective clinical trials currently underway are validating this approach and are accumulating critical evidence to establish ctDNA detection during the MRD phase as a precise biomarker for early prognosis and recurrence risk assessment.

ctDNA detection technologies can be broadly divided into two strategies. The first is a tumor-informed approach, which tracks ctDNA using customized probes designed based on the individual patient's tumor genomic information [1, 10]. For example, Natera's Signatera™ platform creates a personalized panel using ≥16 somatic mutations pre-identified from the patient's primary tumor tissue, and monitors ctDNA in the patient's blood accordingly. Because this method is tailored to each patient, it offers high sensitivity and specificity, greatly enhancing the precision of MRD detection. However, the need for tumor tissue acquisition, the lengthy process, and high costs pose practical limitations.

The second is a tumor-agnostic approach, which utilizes standardized panels that cover major genetic or epigenetic alterations commonly found in specific cancer types [2, 46]. For instance, Guardant Reveal™ and FoundationOne Liquid CDx can be used even when tumor tissue is not available [46]. However, these panels may have lower sensitivity compared to personalized strategies, and there is a risk of missing very low levels of ctDNA, particularly in the MRD setting.

Recently, technologies that distinguish tumor-derived ctDNA from normal cfDNA by analyzing methylation patterns, epigenetic features, and cfDNA fragmentation profiles (fragmentomics) have been developed. Platforms such as cfMeDIP-seq, Galleri™, and DELFI leverage these non-mutation-based approaches to infer tissue of origin, offering a significant advantage [14, 18].

The latest next-generation sequencing (NGS)-based technologies employ ultra-deep sequencing and error suppression techniques to detect even low concentrations of ctDNA [46–48].

However, increased sensitivity also raises the risk of false positives. Clonal hematopoiesis (CH) is a particularly prominent confounding factor [12]. CH refers to the phenomenon in which mutations arising in hematopoietic stem cells lead to the selective expansion of specific cell clones, and it has been reported in approximately 10~20% of adults aged ≥ 70 years [12]. DNMT3A, TET2, and ASXL1 mutations associated with CH can be detected in cfDNA from blood and may be indistinguishable from tumor-derived mutations, which may cause false positives in MRD detection. For example, if CH mutations are misinterpreted as a sign of relapse during MRD monitoring, this may lead to unnecessary anticancer interventions and patient anxiety. In fact, studies on colorectal cancer MRD have shown that some patients with positive ctDNA results were found to have CH-related mutations, and failure to correct for this led to reduced specificity.

To overcome these issues, patient-specific mutation profiling and parallel analysis of white blood cell (WBC) DNA are increasingly being proposed as standard practice [11, 49]. Sequencing WBC-derived DNA allows for the preemptive exclusion of CH mutations, and clinical trials have demonstrated a reduction in false positives. In addition, new ultrasensitive platforms are emerging. For example, PhasED-Seq (phased variant enrichment and detection sequencing) tracks two or more closely located mutations on the same chromosome simultaneously, dramatically reducing background noise. Another example is MAESTRO (minimal allele enrichment through sequencing with targeted recognition oligonucleotides), which enables precise enrichment of ultralow-frequency mutations, allowing detection of VAFs below 0.001% [47]. High-sensitivity technologies such as digital droplet PCR (ddPCR), BEAMing, and deep sequencing also offer superior sensitivity compared to non-targeted sequencing. However, the need for prior information on each patient's tumor mutation spectrum, rigorous discrimination of non-tumor mutations, and consideration of biological variability over long-term follow-up remain major limitations. Ultimately, ctDNA-based MRD detection should not be a mere competition to increase sensitivity, but should evolve toward minimizing false positives while ensuring reproducibility and regulatory reliability. In this process, WBC-matched sequencing, AI-based mutation filtering, and integration of multiple biomarkers are becoming key strategies. Representative methylation-based ctDNA detection platforms include Guardant Reveal, Galleri, and the xM platform developed in China, all of which actively utilize artificial intelligence (AI) and machine learning algorithms to efficiently interpret complex genomic data. Guardant Reveal demonstrated that ctDNA-based MRD detection after surgery in colorectal cancer patients could identify recurrence signals an average of 8–9 months earlier than radiological recurrence, and that MRD positivity was strongly associated with disease-free survival (DFS) and overall survival (OS).

The Galleri platform, originally developed as a multi-cancer early detection (MCED) technology, is now being extended to MRD detection by leveraging tumor-specific methylation patterns. The xM platform, developed in China, reported that MRD-positive patients with colorectal and lung cancer had significantly higher recurrence rates than MRD-negative patients, based on a large cohort of over 10,000 individuals, marking the first large-scale MRD validation study in an East Asian population. Recently, these technological advances have enabled ultrasensitive detection, exemplified by the MAESTRO (minimal allele enrichment through sequencing with targeted recognition oligonucleotides) technology, which has garnered significant attention. MAESTRO effectively enriches large numbers of low-frequency mutations and maintains high accuracy with fewer reads through duplex sequencing. It has been successfully applied to precisely monitor MRD during neoadjuvant chemotherapy in patients with triple-negative breast cancer (TNBC), demonstrating new possibilities for ctDNA-based MRD detection. In contrast, non-targeted NGS-based analyses, such as whole genome sequencing (WGS) or exome sequencing, can comprehensively detect copy number alterations (CNA), point mutations, structural variants, and other genetic abnormalities, and allow ctDNA analysis without prior tumor tissue profiling. However, they require relatively high ctDNA concentrations, and their analytical sensitivity generally remains at the percent level (approximately 1–5%), limiting their use in MRD detection. Low sensitivity limits the clinical application of MRD detection. Therefore, the tumor-agnostic approach is currently considered suitable for exploratory research or for molecular characterization in patients with high tumor burden. In conclusion, despite technological advances, ctDNA-based MRD detection still requires a balance between ultrasensitive detection capability and tailored analytical strategies. The tumor-informed approach enables high sensitivity and specificity by tracking MRD based on the individual tumor's mutational profile, whereas the tumor-agnostic approach has the advantage of being applicable even when tissue samples are unavailable. Future developments are expected to integrate these strategies complementarily and expand toward multi-omics approaches that combine methylation, fragmentomics, and AI-based interpretation. A representative example of the tumor-informed approach is a study that monitored tumor dynamics by measuring circulating tumor DNA (ctDNA) in plasma from colorectal cancer patients with resectable liver metastases [2]. In this study, ctDNA was detected in all 18 patients prior to surgery, and ctDNA levels dropped sharply in most patients after surgery. However, in some patients, ctDNA remained detectable postoperatively, and this group eventually experienced clinical recurrence. Notably, ctDNA provided a signal of recurrence on average 3–5 months earlier than radiological diagnosis. This offered definitive evidence that ctDNA is not merely a marker of residual tumor but a sensitive biomarker that can reflect the risk of recurrence at an early stage. Furthermore, the study demonstrated a close association between treatment response and ctDNA dynamics. Patients whose ctDNA converted to negative after surgery had significantly longer disease-free survival (DFS), whereas those with persistent ctDNA detection postoperatively experienced recurrence within a short period. Thus, ctDNA negativity served as a clinically relevant indicator directly linked to therapeutic efficacy. This study is regarded as the first clinical demonstration of the concept of MRD monitoring using ctDNA. In particular, it provided clinical evidence supporting the validity of the tumor-informed approach and showed that ctDNA can predict tumor recurrence earlier than imaging or conventional tumor markers. Numerous subsequent MRD studies in colorectal, breast, and lung cancers have all built upon the conceptual foundation established by this research. In this context, the prospective clinical trial PRODIGE-14 (NCT01442935, phase II) evaluated treatment response by serially measuring ctDNA during preoperative systemic therapy in colorectal cancer patients with potentially resectable liver metastases [42, 50]. ctDNA was measured at three time points: baseline (treatment initiation), 4 weeks after treatment, and immediately before surgery. In this study, droplet digital PCR was used to analyze KRAS mutations in ctDNA, and the detection sensitivity at baseline was very high at 91% ($N = 42/46$). Notably, patients with persistent KRAS ctDNA detection after 4 weeks of therapy had a significantly lower rate of liver metastasis resection, and those with detectable ctDNA immediately before surgery had shorter overall survival (OS). These results suggest that monitoring ctDNA dynamics during treatment may help assess the suitability of hepatic resection and predict prognosis in colorectal cancer patients with limited liver metastases. A similar approach has been applied in early breast cancer patients [10]. After profiling somatic mutations in the primary tumor using next-generation sequencing (NGS), personalized digital PCR-based ctDNA analysis was performed to serially monitor tumor-specific ctDNA in the patient's plasma. The study included 101 early breast cancer patients, who were followed long-term after surgery and standard adjuvant therapy. ctDNA monitoring was initiated immediately after completion of treatment (baseline) and subsequently performed at regular 3-month intervals during follow-up. The results showed that detection of ctDNA after treatment was significantly associated with recurrence compared to those without detectable ctDNA (HR = 25.1, $p < 0.001$). In 89% of patients who experienced recurrence, ctDNA was detected on average 10.7 months (range: 0.7–24 months) prior to clinical relapse. Notably, among ctDNA-positive patients, the cumulative incidence of relapse reached 89% at 3 years of follow-up, whereas ctDNA-negative patients demonstrated a 3-year disease-free survival (DFS) rate of 93%, confirming the clinical value of negative predictive power.

Multivariate analysis also identified ctDNA positivity as an independent predictor of recurrence, and it remained a strong prognostic factor even after adjusting for established clinicopathological variables (such as TNM stage and HR/HER2 status). These findings demonstrate that serial ctDNA-based monitoring is effective for MRD assessment and early detection of recurrence in patients with early breast cancer, suggesting the potential for preemptive therapeutic intervention before clinical relapse. Furthermore, this study strongly supports the use of ctDNA monitoring as an early warning signal prior to clinical recurrence, facilitating personalized treatment planning and follow-up strategies for patients.

Signatera is a tumor-informed ctDNA analysis platform that enables precise monitoring of blood ctDNA based on more than 16 unique somatic mutations pre-identified from each patient's tumor tissue. This system is primarily focused on tracking MRD after surgery or standard therapy and on the early detection of recurrence risk.

In a representative study, patients with stage II and III colorectal cancer underwent regular blood sampling after completion of therapy, and the Signatera assay was performed. The results showed that patients with ctDNA positivity had a significantly higher risk of recurrence compared to ctDNA-negative patients, and recurrence could be predicted on average 8.7 months earlier than radiological diagnosis [30]. Particularly, in the context of adjuvant chemotherapy decision-making, ctDNA-positive patients derived substantial benefit from treatment, while ctDNA-negative patients were provided with evidence to avoid unnecessary therapy.

The clinical rationale for this personalized ctDNA-based approach was conceptually supported by the TRACERx study [1]. The TRACERx study profiled the entire tumor genome in more than 100 patients with early-stage non-small cell lung cancer (NSCLC) after surgery and conducted patient-specific ctDNA monitoring. The study demonstrated that ctDNA detection was closely associated with recurrence risk and could capture recurrence signals up to 11 months earlier than imaging-based diagnosis. In particular, ctDNA-positive patients had significantly lower disease-free survival (DFS), and ctDNA clearance was directly linked to long-term prognosis, thereby establishing tumor-informed ctDNA monitoring as a powerful biomarker for MRD detection and recurrence prediction.

Subsequent clinical validation of Signatera was expanded to cohorts of breast and colorectal cancer patients, confirming the clinical utility of ctDNA-based MRD analysis for early relapse detection and treatment decision support, respectively. In addition, Signatera has been applied in clinical studies for MRD assessment across various solid tumors, including breast, lung, and bladder cancers, playing a key role in the development of personalized treatment strategies and long-term follow-up. It has been designated as a Breakthrough Device by the FDA in 2019, recognizing the potential clinical value of this technology.

In conclusion, Signatera is a leading ctDNA analysis platform for the implementation of MRD-based precision medicine, demonstrating excellent performance in MRD assessment, recurrence prediction, and treatment guidance. Ongoing clinical evidence, including the TRACERx study, continues to reinforce its value.

TARDIS (targeted digital sequencing) is an ultrasensitive method for detecting minimal amounts of plasma ctDNA. It is a next-generation targeted digital sequencing technology developed for the highly sensitive detection of minimal residual disease (MRD) DNA. Conventional ctDNA detection methods typically target fewer than several dozen mutations; however, TARDIS employs a patient-specific (tumor-informed) approach, enabling the simultaneous targeting of up to 100–115 unique mutations derived from each individual's tumor. This broad targeting strategy allows for the accumulation and integrated analysis of low-frequency variants, resulting in approximately 100-fold greater sensitivity compared to existing methods. The technological core lies in the combination of ultra-deep sequencing and advanced error suppression techniques. Thanks to these features, TARDIS is effectively utilized for real-time monitoring of therapeutic response during neoadjuvant therapy and for the early detection of residual disease following treatment completion. In particular, it is gaining attention as an innovative platform that significantly enhances the reliability of MRD assessment and recurrence prediction in high-risk patient groups, such as those with triple-negative breast cancer (TNBC). In a representative study, serial longitudinal analyses were conducted on 33 patients with stage I–III early breast cancer, with a total of 80 plasma samples collected. Up to 115 tumor-specific mutations were selected as targets for each patient to enable precise ctDNA tracking. At the pretreatment stage, TARDIS detected ctDNA in all patients, with a reported median allele frequency (AF) of 0.11%. After completion of neoadjuvant therapy, patients who achieved a pathological complete response (pathCR) exhibited a marked reduction in ctDNA concentration, with a significant difference in median AF compared to those with residual disease (0.003% vs. 0.017%, $p = 0.0057$). The diagnostic performance of TARDIS was evaluated with an area under the curve (AUC) of 0.83, demonstrating a high level of molecular response assessment capability. Furthermore, the magnitude of ctDNA reduction during neoadjuvant therapy was more pronounced in patients who achieved pathCR, suggesting that TARDIS can be effectively utilized for monitoring therapeutic response and evaluating residual disease. This study demonstrated that personalized ctDNA analysis can reflect a patient's treatment course in real time and emphasized that the TARDIS platform can play a pivotal role in MRD detection and recurrence prediction as an innovative tool for precision medicine. In colorectal cancer, the DYNAMIC trial and the GALAXY cohort study of CIRCULATE-Japan provide representative clinical evidence. The DYNAMIC trial was a randomized prospective clinical study that evaluated the clinical efficacy of a ctDNA-based personalized treatment strategy in 455 patients with stage II colorectal cancer [26]. In the study design, patients were divided into two groups. One group determined the need for adjuvant chemotherapy (ACT) based on conventional standard criteria (pathological risk factors), while the other group adjusted treatment plans according to ctDNA levels measured at 4 and 7 weeks post-surgery. Patients with positive ctDNA were recommended to receive adjuvant chemotherapy, whereas those with negative ctDNA omitted treatment. The results showed that in the ctDNA-guided group, only 15% of patients received adjuvant chemotherapy, compared to 28% in the standard care group—effectively halving the rate. Nevertheless, the 2-year disease-free survival (DFS) was 93.5% in the ctDNA group and 92.4% in the standard group, demonstrating non-inferiority. Furthermore, 5-year follow-up data revealed no significant differences in overall survival (OS) or recurrence rates between the two groups. These findings indicate that a ctDNA-based personalized strategy can safely reduce unnecessary chemotherapy while preserving patient outcomes. Thus, the DYNAMIC trial is regarded as a pioneering study demonstrating that ctDNA-based MRD monitoring can serve as a guideline in actual treatment decision-making, marking a turning point in the era of precision medicine for colorectal cancer.

The GALAXY trial, published in 2024 as part of the CIRCULATE-Japan project, was a prospective observational study that enrolled 2240 patients with resectable stage II and III colorectal cancer [27]. The study aimed to assess ctDNA positivity at defined postoperative intervals (e.g., 4 weeks after surgery) using a tumor-informed ctDNA assay, and to use these results both to guide adjuvant chemotherapy decisions and to predict recurrence risk. The results showed that approximately 20% of all patients were ctDNA-positive after surgery, and among these, 78.3% experienced recurrence during the follow-up period. By contrast, the recurrence rate in the ctDNA-negative group was only 13.1%, confirming ctDNA negativity as a strong prognostic indicator. Notably, adjuvant chemotherapy in ctDNA-positive patients conferred significant therapeutic benefit, particularly in terms of improved disease-free survival (DFS). Furthermore, the GALAXY trial demonstrated that recurrence signals could be detected more than 8 months earlier on average compared to radiological diagnosis. These findings underscore the value of early intervention and indicate that ctDNA-based MRD detection can serve as a pivotal decision-making tool, extending beyond recurrence prediction to actual treatment stratification. In summary, the DYNAMIC trial demonstrated that ctDNA can serve as a reliable basis for modulating treatment intensity, while the GALAXY trial established that ctDNA positivity is a strong independent predictor of recurrence risk in a large patient cohort. Both studies provide critical evidence supporting ctDNA-based MRD monitoring as a precision medicine tool that enables both the avoidance of unnecessary treatment and the implementation of early intervention strategies in colorectal cancer patients. Various clinical studies related to MRD detection have demonstrated the clinical utility of liquid biopsy technologies based on CTCs and ctDNA. In particular, prospective studies targeting major solid tumors such as colorectal, breast, and lung cancers have repeatedly confirmed that MRD status is closely associated with the risk of recurrence. In the field of breast cancer, the ChemoNEAR study and the TBCRC 030 trial provide representative evidence. The ChemoNEAR study evaluated the clinical feasibility of MRD detection and recurrence risk prediction in early breast cancer patients using NeXT Personal, an ultrasensitive whole-genome sequencing-based tumor-informed ctDNA platform. In this study, plasma samples were repeatedly collected from a total of 76 patients at diagnosis, during neoadjuvant chemotherapy (NAC), after surgery, and throughout the follow-up period for ctDNA analysis. The results showed that MRD was detected in 100% of patients who experienced recurrence, with ctDNA being identified on average 12.5 months (up to 2 years) earlier than clinical recurrence. Conversely, none of the patients who remained ctDNA-negative during follow-up experienced recurrence. These findings indicate that the high negative predictive value (NPV) of ctDNA can help reduce unnecessary treatment, while early identification and intensive management of ctDNA-positive patients is also possible. In other words, the ChemoNEAR study provides empirical evidence that ctDNA is a precision medicine tool capable of supporting both risk stratification and treatment intensity decisions. The TBCRC 030 trial was a case-control study conducted in patients with triple-negative breast cancer (TNBC) receiving neoadjuvant chemotherapy, utilizing MAESTRO (minimal allele enrichment through sequencing with targeted recognition oligonucleotides), a highly sensitive mutation enrichment sequencing technique, to analyze the correlation between ctDNA tumor fraction (TFx) and residual cancer burden (RCB) [51]. Plasma samples were collected at baseline, week 3, and week 12 (end of treatment), and up to 1000 mutations were tracked in a total of 114 plasma samples using personalized ctDNA analysis. The results showed that in the responder group (RCB 0/1), ctDNA TFx decreased by 285-fold, whereas in the non-responder group (RCB 2/3), the decrease was only 24-fold. In addition, at week 12, the ctDNA Clearance rate was closely associated with RCB grade, and in 83% (5/6) of relapsed patients, ctDNA continued to be detected at the end of treatment. In 58% of patients, ctDNA TFx decreased below the detection limit of conventional commercial assays, underscoring the need for ultrasensitive platforms. This study demonstrated that dynamic changes in ctDNA are effective indicators for evaluating NAC response and predicting recurrence risk. It also showed the potential of MRD monitoring to serve simultaneously as a biomarker of response and a prognostic biomarker. However, the study is limited by a small sample size and its restriction to the TNBC subtype, highlighting the need for validation in larger cohorts and across diverse molecular subtypes. In lung cancer (NSCLC), the TRACERx study and IMpower010 trial have demonstrated the potential of MRD-based precision medicine [1]. As previously described, the TRACERx study showed that post-surgical ctDNA monitoring enables early detection of recurrence. The IMpower010 trial is a phase III clinical study evaluating the efficacy of adjuvant immunotherapy (atezolizumab) after surgery in patients with resectable stage IB–IIIA NSCLC. According to retrospective ctDNA analysis in this study, patients whose ctDNA converted to negative immediately after treatment had significantly prolonged disease-free survival (DFS). Conversely, patients with persistently positive ctDNA after adjuvant therapy had a markedly higher risk of recurrence, suggesting that dynamic changes in ctDNA may reflect immunotherapy responsiveness. Notably, ctDNA clearance functioned as a strong biomarker for predicting patient prognosis independently of conventional clinical and pathological factors, and demonstrated clinical value as a tool for identifying patients who would benefit from adjuvant immunotherapy. In addition, the clinical utility of ctDNA-based MRD detection continues to be reported in various cancers, including bladder, pancreatic, and gastric cancers. For example, in bladder cancer, post-surgical ctDNA positivity was associated with increased risk of recurrence, and in pancreatic and gastric cancers, ctDNA monitoring after surgery and chemotherapy provided important clues for early detection of recurrence and personalized therapeutic intervention. This body of evidence indicates that ctDNA-based MRD assessment is becoming a central pillar of posttreatment patient management across cancer types. As described above, CTC- and ctDNA-based MRD detection technologies are becoming essential tools for the realization of precision medicine. However, there remain significant challenges, including low sensitivity and specificity, high costs, and complex analytical processes. For instance, even with ultrasensitive technologies, ctDNA detection reliability can be compromised at extremely low variant allele frequencies (VAFs), and CTCs, due to their rarity in blood, are susceptible to technical variability during isolation. These limitations introduce uncertainty in clinical interpretation and ultimately raise concerns about the reliability of patient-specific therapeutic decision-making. Consequently, future research is expanding toward multi-omics-based analyses and integrated data interpretation using AI algorithms. Rather than relying on a single-analyte, integrating analyses of ctDNA mutations and methylation patterns, CTC proteomic and transcriptomic signals, and EV-based miRNA and protein signatures can offset individual limitations and maximize strengths. In particular, machine learning and deep learning-based AI approaches are essential for efficient interpretation of high-dimensional big data. Some studies have already reported attempts to integrate ctDNA and EV data to enhance the sensitivity of MRD detection, which may provide a solution to the issue of reproducibility in clinical settings. Notably, extracellular vesicles (EVs) are rapidly emerging as a novel analyte for MRD detection. EVs are carriers of biological information selectively secreted by tumor cells, encapsulating and protecting a variety of molecules (proteins, miRNA, lncRNA, DNA fragments, etc.) within a stable lipid bilayer. These characteristics allow EVs to survive relatively longer in the bloodstream and stably carry tumor-specific signatures, offering the potential to overcome the limitations of conventional CTC- or ctDNA-based approaches. In fact, early clinical studies have reported attempts to detect MRD status or predict recurrence at an early stage by combining miRNA and protein panels within EVs. However, EV-based MRD detection remains in the early stages of research, with major obstacles including the lack of standardized isolation and purification technologies and unresolved issues regarding the reproducibility of EV cargo analysis. Although various methods such as ultracentrifugation, chromatography, and immunoaffinity separation are employed, there is no internationally agreed standard regarding reproducibility, purity, and cost-effectiveness required for clinical application. Furthermore, the reproducibility of molecular contents within EVs and the lack of effective methods to distinguish tumor-specific EVs from background (non-tumor) EVs remain challenges to be addressed. For future advancement, the following are necessary: (1) international standardization of EV isolation and characterization, (2) demonstration of clinical validity through large-scale prospective clinical trials, (3) data sharing among multiple institutions and establishment of AI-based interpretation platforms, and (4) development of multiparametric MRD assessment models integrating EVs, ctDNA, and CTCs. With these foundations in place, EVs could establish themselves as a third MRD analyte complementing existing ctDNA and CTCs, ultimately contributing to the achievement of truly personalized therapy and recurrence prevention in clinical practice.

5.3 Companion Diagnosis

Companion diagnosis (CDx) is a precision medicine approach that predicts the likelihood of response to a specific therapy based on the molecular biological characteristics of a patient's tumor and is performed alongside treatment decision-making to ensure the safety and efficacy of the corresponding treatment [3]. It goes beyond a simple auxiliary test, forming the core of the drug–diagnostic codevelopment model in which therapeutics and diagnostics are inextricably linked throughout anticancer drug development and clinical application (Fig. 5.4).

The concept of CDx was formally established in 1998, when the HercepTest™ (Dako) and PathVysion® HER-2 DNA Probe Kit (Abbott/Vysis) received FDA approval for use in HER2-positive breast cancer patients undergoing trastuzumab (Herceptin®) therapy. This was the first regulatory approval linking a single drug to a single biomarker, marking the advent of the precision oncology paradigm. As a result, only patients with HER2 overexpression or gene amplification were eligible for trastuzumab treatment, thereby introducing the practical implementation of "patient selection-based personalized therapy" into clinical reality.

Subsequently, with the development of targeted therapies against various molecular targets such as EGFR, ALK, ROS1, BRAF, NTRK, and RET, companion diagnostics have become an essential component of anticancer treatment strategies [3]. The FDA defines companion diagnostics as "medical devices that are essential for the safe and effective use of a specific drug," and thus, CDx not only detects biomarkers but also defines the population eligible for therapy while excluding unsuitable patients. This enables the provision of individualized treatment, reducing unnecessary side effects and costs, and provides the basis for maximizing therapeutic efficacy in both clinical trials and real-world practice.

In particular, liquid biopsy-based companion diagnostics are emerging as a crucial alternative when tissue biopsy is not feasible or tumor heterogeneity is pronounced. For example, the detection of the EGFR T790M mutation in ctDNA to determine eligibility for third-generation tyrosine kinase inhibitor (TKI) osimertinib therapy is already widely used in clinical practice and has been approved by the FDA. In addition, blood-based assessment of biomarkers such as MSI-H (microsatellite instability-high) and TMB (tumor mutational burden) is being used to predict indications for immunotherapy [46]. This approach is increasingly being integrated into clinical practice. These changes clearly demonstrate that the analytes for CDx are no longer limited to tissue, but are expanding to include liquid biopsy-based ctDNA, CTCs, EVs, and others. In summary, CDx serves both as a gateway to cancer therapy and as a key to enabling personalized treatment. Initially, it was limited to single biomarker-based tests linked to specific drugs, but its scope has now expanded to include multi-biomarker panels, next-generation sequencing (NGS)-based integrated diagnostics, and liquid biopsy-based precision diagnostics. This evolution goes beyond mere technological advancement; it also solidifies a co-development ecosystem for drug and diagnostic platform development from regulatory science and industrial perspectives. Traditional tissue biopsy has long been the standard analytical method for companion diagnostics (CDx). Cells and DNA obtained directly from tumor tissue have provided the most reliable evidence for determining drug responsiveness, and the clinical introduction of various targeted therapies such as HER2, EGFR, BRAF,

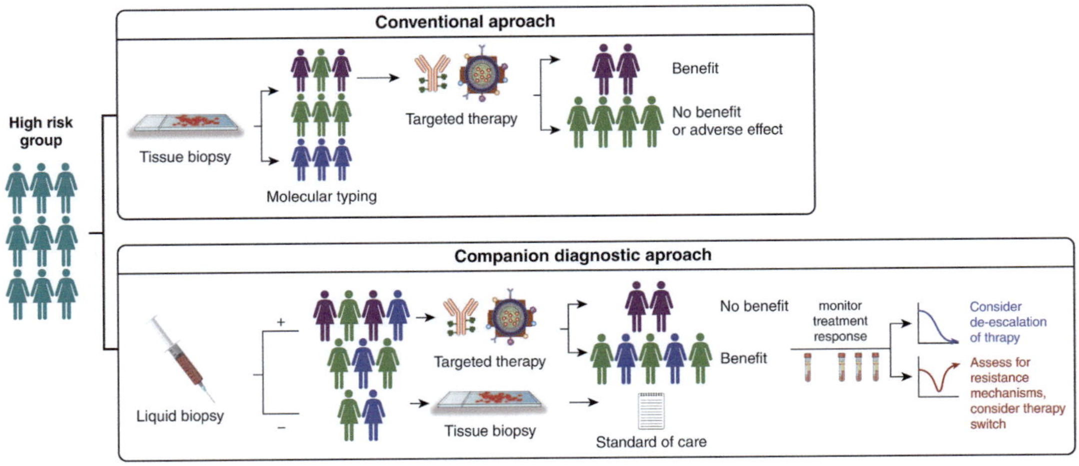

Fig. 5.4 Liquid biopsy for companion diagnosis

ALK, and ROS1 would not have been possible without tissue-based CDx. However, in real-world clinical settings, repeated tissue sampling is often challenging due to the anatomical location of the tumor, the patient's overall condition, and procedural risks. Furthermore, the spatial and temporal heterogeneity characteristic of solid tumors has raised ongoing concerns that a single-tissue sample may not represent the entire disease. In this context, liquid biopsy (LB) has emerged as a new tool to complement or replace tissue-based CDx. In particular, liquid biopsy using circulating tumor DNA (ctDNA) offers the advantages of being noninvasive and allowing for repeated sampling, thereby enabling real-time monitoring of tumor genetic changes in patients. This approach provides critical information for early adjustment of personalized treatment strategies by capturing newly emerging resistance mutations or clonal evolution during therapy. Moreover, even in situations where tissue sampling is impossible or carries significant risk, it allows for the detection of biomarkers related to therapeutic response, facilitating the rapid identification of new actionable targets. In fact, these possibilities are being realized through regulatory approvals. Notably, the Cobas® EGFR Mutation Test v2, which can detect EGFR mutations, especially the T790M resistance mutation, is one of the first FDA-approved tests available for both tissue-based and blood-based ctDNA samples. This test is used to determine the administration of the third-generation TKI osimertinib in patients with metastatic non-small cell lung cancer (NSCLC), and by providing a noninvasive alternative for patients in whom tissue sampling is not feasible, it has broadened the scope of clinical application. This approval marks an important milestone, demonstrating that liquid biopsy has entered the realm of companion diagnostics directly linked to therapeutic decision-making, beyond being merely a research tool. However, there are still limitations that must be addressed before liquid biopsy-based CDx can become a clinical standard. The most prominent issue is the limitation in sensitivity. While ctDNA-based liquid biopsy tests generally exhibit high specificity, they may fail to detect mutations when ctDNA concentrations are extremely low. This can lead to false negative results, posing the risk of inappropriate exclusion of patients from treatment. Particularly in situations such as pretreatment or post-surgical minimal residual disease (MRD), where blood ctDNA levels are extremely low, a negative result does not necessarily indicate the absence of mutations—an important caution for clinicians. In fact, current clinical guidelines recommend tissue rebiopsy and additional molecular analysis if a negative result is obtained from a blood-based test. Significant technological advances are being made to overcome the sensitivity issue. Highly sensitive techniques such as digital droplet PCR (ddPCR), BEAMing, and ultra-deep next-generation sequencing (ultra-deep NGS) enable detection of trace amounts of ctDNA, with some assays capable of identifying variant allele frequencies (VAFs) as low as 0.1% [2, 48]. However, despite these technological advances, the challenge of reliably detecting extremely low VAFs while simultaneously minimizing false positives remains unresolved. Ultimately, liquid biopsy-based CDx complements traditional tissue-based diagnostics by leveraging its inherent advantages of noninvasiveness and repeatability. In particular, it offers a new diagnostic paradigm that can reflect real-time tumor evolution, especially in cases of recurrence and therapeutic resistance. Nevertheless, technical standardization and large-scale clinical validation are essential to overcome the risk of false negatives due to low sensitivity. In the future, the integration of multi-analyte approaches, AI-based data interpretation, and the establishment of international guidelines will be necessary for liquid biopsy to become a clinical standard that supplements or replaces tissue biopsy in the CDx field. In the early stages of companion diagnostics (CDx) development, the mainstream approach was to detect single gene mutations to predict specific drug responses. Representative examples of single-gene-based companion diagnostic platforms include the Cobas® EGFR Mutation Test v2 (EGFR single gene mutation), therascreen PIK3CA RGQ PCR Kit (PIK3CA single-gene mutation), and Resolution ctDx FIRST. While these platforms offer the advantage of accurately detecting a single gene mutation with a clear association to targeted therapies, they are limited by their focus on only one gene mutation, which introduces the possibility of false negatives and makes it difficult to capture complex mutations or tumor heterogeneity. Therefore, alongside considerations of false negative risk, the need for transitioning to multi-gene panel-based assays will also be discussed (Table 5.1).

5.3.1 Cobas® EGFR Mutation Test v2

The Cobas® EGFR Mutation Test v2 is a real-time PCR-based companion diagnostic platform developed for the qualitative detection of epidermal growth factor receptor (EGFR) gene mutations in patients with non-small cell lung cancer (NSCLC). This assay is designed to analyze both formalin-fixed paraffin-embedded tissue (FFPET) and plasma-derived cfDNA from EDTA-treated blood, making it applicable to both tissue and blood-based specimens [52]. In NSCLC treatment, EGFR tyrosine kinase inhibitors (TKIs) such as erlotinib and gefitinib have demonstrated remarkable efficacy; however, approximately 90% of patients eventually develop resistance during the course of therapy. The most common resistance mechanism is the T790M mutation in EGFR exon 20, which is known to cause loss of efficacy of first-generation TKIs [6]. The Cobas® EGFR Mutation Test v2 addresses this clinical need by enabling early, noninvasive, real-time detection of the T790M mutation, thereby providing critical information for therapeutic strategy adjustment, particularly regarding the use of third-generation EGFR TKIs such as TAGRISSO™ (osimertinib). Clinical validation studies have shown that this assay achieved a PPA of 95.9%, NPA of 99.7%, and OPA of 98.8% for EGFR exon 19 deletion detection. For the L858R mutation, the PPA was 90.6%, NPA 98.6%, and OPA 97.5%. For the T790M mutation (based on the AURA2 clinical trial), the PPA was 88.3%, NPA 97.3%, and OPA 91.0%, demonstrating high accuracy even in blood-based testing. The analytical sensitivity of assay has been reported to enable detection of variants at allele frequencies as low as ~5%, with low cross-reactivity and high reproducibility. The Cobas® EGFR Mutation Test v2 offers clinical value beyond simple mutation detection. It is used not only to determine eligibility for targeted therapies such as TARCEVA® (erlotinib) and TAGRISSO™ (osimertinib) based on EGFR mutation status, but also for investigational use in monitoring post-surgical recurrence and tracking resistance mutations during treatment in clinical

Table 5.1 Targeted gene-based liquid biopsy CDx platforms

Platform	Target genes/ biomarkers	Indication	Sample type	Technology	Regulatory status	Strengths	Limitations
Cobas® EGFR Mutation Test v2	EGFR (exon 19 del, L858R, T790M)	NSCLC	Tissue, plasma	Real-time PCR	FDA CDx (USA)	Detects key resistance mutations (e.g., T790M), high accuracy	Limited to EGFR; false negatives at low VAF
Therascreen® PIK3CA RGQ PCR Kit	PIK3CA (11 mutations)	HR+/ HER2− breast cancer	Tissue, plasma	Real-time PCR	FDA CDx (USA) CE-IVD (EU)	Selects PIQRAY®-eligible patients, validated by the SOLAR-1 trial	Rebiopsy needed if plasma is negative
Resolution ctDx FIRST	KRAS G12C	NSCLC	Plasma	Hybrid-capture NGS	FDA CDx (USA) (adagrasib)	Effective noninvasive KRAS G12C detection	Needs a confirmatory tissue test if negative

research settings. The advantages of blood-based liquid biopsy are particularly significant for patients in whom tissue sampling is difficult or repeated assessments are required, highlighting its clinical utility as a complementary or alternative diagnostic tool to tissue biopsy. The FDA has officially approved the Cobas® EGFR Mutation Test v2 as a companion diagnostic (CDx) device, representing a notable example that demonstrates how liquid biopsy-based companion diagnostics are approaching the clinical gold standard in tumor molecular diagnostics. This assay serves as a key tool enabling the implementation of precision medicine throughout the management of NSCLC patients by detecting EGFR mutations.

5.3.2 Therascreen PIK3CA RGQ PCR Kit

The therascreen® PIK3CA RGQ PCR Kit (QIAGEN) is a real-time quantitative PCR assay developed as an in vitro diagnostic (IVD) for the detection of PIK3CA mutations in patients with hormone receptor-positive (HR-positive), HER2-negative advanced breast cancer [53]. This assay is designed to analyze both formalin-fixed paraffin-embedded tissue (FFPET) and circulating tumor DNA (ctDNA) isolated from plasma. The plasma-based testing option expands clinical applicability by providing a complementary alternative for patients in whom invasive tissue biopsy is challenging, although tissue testing is still recommended in plasma-negative cases [54, 55]. The intended use of this test is to identify HR-positive/HER2-negative breast cancer patients and determine their eligibility for treatment with the PIK3CA inhibitor PIQRAY® (alpelisib) in combination with fulvestrant.

The therascreen® PIK3CA RGQ PCR Kit targets a total of 11 PIK3CA mutations. The main mutation sites include Exon 7 (C420R), Exon 9 (E542K, E545A, E545D [1635G > T], E545G, E545K, Q546E, Q546R), and Exon 20 (H1047L, H1047R, H1047Y). These are major hotspots within the PIK3CA gene, known to aberrantly activate the PI3K/AKT signaling pathway in tumor cells, thereby promoting cell growth and survival. In particular, these mutations are well established to be closely associated with endocrine therapy resistance and poor prognosis in HR+/HER2− breast cancer patients.

Detection of PIK3CA mutations in blood offers the advantage of noninvasively guiding patient treatment decisions. However, as the possibility of false-negative results cannot be excluded when mutations are not detected in plasma, a repeat FFPET tissue-based test is recommended for patients with negative plasma results. This approach maximizes diagnostic sensitivity.

The clinical validity of the therascreen® PIK3CA RGQ PCR Kit was demonstrated in the SOLAR-1 clinical trial (NCT02437318). This phase III randomized trial evaluated the efficacy of alpelisib (PIQRAY®) in combination with fulvestrant in patients with HR+/HER2− advanced breast cancer harboring PIK3CA mutations who had progressed on prior endocrine therapy. In the SOLAR-1 study, the progression-free survival (PFS) in the alpelisib-fulvestrant group was 11.0 months (95% CI, 7.5–14.5), showing a significant improvement compared to 5.7 months (95% CI, 3.7–7.4) in the placebo group (HR = 0.65, $p < 0.001$). This provides strong evidence supporting the clinical benefit of PI3Kα inhibitor therapy in patients with PIK3CA mutations.

Furthermore, subsequent analyses of SOLAR-1 demonstrated that patient identification based solely on plasma ctDNA analysis was clinically comparable to tissue-based analysis. Patients with PIK3CA mutations detected in plasma-based ctDNA also experienced PFS extension with alpelisib treatment, comparable to those with tissue-based mutation positivity, thereby firmly establishing the potential of noninvasive liquid biopsy-based companion diagnostics.

In addition, the SOLAR-1 study reported positive results in terms of overall survival (OS). Among patients with metastatic disease, the median survival was 37.2 months (95% CI, 28.7–43.6) in the alpelisib-fulvestrant group, compared to 22.8 months (95% CI, 19.0–26.8) in the placebo-fulvestrant group (HR = 0.68, 95%

CI, 0.46–1.00). Notably, similar trends were observed in the subgroup of patients with prior chemotherapy experience, suggesting that PIQRAY® may provide survival benefits across diverse patient populations.

In conclusion, the therascreen® PIK3CA RGQ PCR Kit enables rapid and accurate assessment of PIK3CA mutation status in patients with HR+/HER2− advanced breast cancer, thereby facilitating the administration of alpelisib. The ability to detect plasma-based ctDNA offers utility even in clinical situations where tissue access is challenging, demonstrating that liquid biopsy-based companion diagnostics can serve as a key tool for implementing precision medicine in real-world clinical practice.

5.3.3 Resolution Bioscience Resolution ctDx FIRST

Resolution ctDx FIRST (Resolution Bioscience) is a liquid biopsy-based companion diagnostic (CDx) platform developed for the noninvasive detection of KRAS G12C mutations in patients with non-small cell lung cancer (NSCLC) [56, 57]. This assay extracts circulating cell-free DNA (cfDNA) from plasma and applies hybrid capture-based next-generation sequencing (NGS) to identify target gene mutations. Jointly developed by Resolution Bioscience and Agilent, it received premarket approval (PMA: P210040) from the US FDA in December 2022 as a companion diagnostic for detecting KRAS G12C mutations for KRAZATI™ (adagrasib) therapy [58].

The primary objective of Resolution Bioscience's Resolution ctDx FIRST is to rapidly and accurately identify NSCLC patients with KRAS G12C mutations to assess their eligibility for adagrasib treatment. At the time of approval, the FDA particularly noted the value of Resolution ctDx FIRST as a noninvasive alternative for patients in whom tissue samples are difficult to obtain. Although the current CDx indication is limited to KRAS G12C mutations, this assay platform is technically capable of detecting other key mutations such as EGFR exon 19 deletion, L858R, and T790M, although its FDA-approved indication is currently limited to KRAS G12C.

In analytical performance validation, Resolution ctDx FIRST demonstrated high accuracy, with a positive percent agreement (PPA) of 96.2%, negative percent agreement (NPA) of 98%, and a false positive rate of 0% in concordance studies with an external ddPCR-based reference method. Furthermore, clinical validity was confirmed through bridging analysis using plasma samples from the KRYSTAL-1 clinical trial. Among 47 patients identified as KRAS G12C-positive by Resolution ctDx FIRST, the objective response rate (ORR) was 51.1% (95% CI: 36.1–65.9%), consistent with the ORR of 42.9% (95% CI: 33.5–52.6%) reported in the original adagrasib clinical cohort. These data demonstrate the assay's ability to link diagnosis with therapeutic response, supporting its effectiveness as a patient selection tool in clinical practice.

The clinical value of Resolution ctDx FIRST is particularly evident in patient populations where tissue biopsy is not feasible or is insufficient. It complements conventional tissue-based testing and can be utilized as a precision diagnostic tool to support personalized treatment decisions [4, 5]. However, the plasma–tissue concordance rate for KRAS G12C mutation detection remains at approximately 61%, indicating that reflex tissue testing is still necessary for patients with negative blood test results.

In conclusion, Resolution ctDx FIRST represents a recent FDA-approved liquid biopsy-based CDx technology that effectively identifies patients eligible for adagrasib therapy through KRAS G12C mutation detection. As a highly sensitive and specific diagnostic platform, it addresses the limitations of tissue-based diagnostics and offers the potential for expansion to a broader range of target genes. Moreover, this case illustrates both the achievements and limitations of single-gene-based CDx, marking an important turning point that explains the growing interest in NGS-based multigene panel strategies in current clinical practice.

In summary, single-gene-based companion diagnostic platforms have provided a simple and intuitive "1 drug–1 biomarker–1 test" model by precisely detecting biomarkers directly linked to specific drugs. This was a significant achievement in the early stages of precision medicine, enabling the co-development of therapeutics and diagnostics, with landmark examples such as trastuzumab–HER2, EGFR TKI–EGFR mutation, and alpelisib–PIK3CA mutation transforming the paradigm of cancer therapy. However, such single-gene models do not fully capture the complex molecular heterogeneity of cancer or the simultaneous occurrence of multiple mutations, and are limited in their ability to detect acquired resistance mutations in real time during treatment.

In this context, next-generation sequencing (NGS)-based multigene panels have recently attracted significant attention. Multigene panel testing enables the simultaneous detection of various types of genetic alterations—including single-nucleotide variants (SNVs), copy number alterations (CNAs), insertions and deletions (indels), and gene fusions—within a single panel. In particular, NGS-based multigene panel assays targeting circulating tumor DNA (cfDNA) in plasma allow for comprehensive, noninvasive acquisition of tumor genetic information. This approach can contribute to clinical decision-making even in patients with high tumor heterogeneity or in situations where tissue samples are difficult to obtain. Notably, FoundationOne Liquid CDx and Guardant360 CDx are both FDA-approved multigene panel platforms, capable of simultaneously analyzing over 300 and 50 gene alterations, respectively, and are approved as companion diagnostics for a variety of therapeutics. Additionally, the Oncomine Dx Target Test is approved for the detection of EGFR, ALK, ROS1, and BRAF mutations in NSCLC and can be used with both tissue and blood samples. Thus, multigene panel-based CDx enables comprehensive genomic profiling (CGP), which was not possible with single biomarker approaches, thereby expanding the foundation for precision medicine in clinical practice. However, there are practical limitations. NGS-based testing is costly, and the interpretation of results often encounters variants of uncertain significance (VUS), where the clinical relevance of detected alterations is unclear. Furthermore, in patients with extremely low cfDNA concentrations, the risk of false negatives remains, and insurance coverage and regulatory approval vary significantly by country. Nevertheless, NGS-based multigene panel diagnostics are regarded as a key technology in the transition from single-biomarker approaches to multi-biomarker precision medicine. The following section will review representative NGS-based multigene panel platforms and discuss in detail how they contribute to the implementation of precision medicine. The various platforms introduced below are designed for comprehensive genomic profiling (CGP) based on the simultaneous analysis of multiple genes; some are for research use only (RUO), while others are clinically applied through CLIA-certified laboratories (LDTs). Although all aim to advance precision medicine, only a limited number have received official FDA CDx approval (Table 5.2).

5.3.4 Archer Reveal ctDNA 28 (28 Genes)

Archer Reveal ctDNA™ 28 is an NGS-based liquid biopsy platform designed to simultaneously detect 28 key gene alterations commonly found across solid tumors from circulating tumor DNA (cfDNA) in plasma [4, 5, 59]. This system utilizes Anchored Multiplex PCR (AMP) technology, attaching unique molecular identifiers (UMIs) to individual DNA fragments, followed by ultra-deep sequencing, thereby optimizing detection of even ultralow-frequency variants [48, 60]. Target genes include EGFR, ALK, ROS1, BRAF, MET, and PIK3CA, among others, with many alterations directly linked to therapeutic targets in non-small cell lung cancer (NSCLC) patients [4, 61]. The clinical performance of Archer Reveal ctDNA™ 28 has been validated in multiple studies. In a study of NSCLC patients undergoing plasma-based NGS testing, ctDNA alterations were detected in 64.3% of cases, and among patients with confirmed driver mutations, the concordance rate between tissue and plasma was 96.1%. Based on these findings, treatment strategies were altered in 21.9% of patients, with

Table 5.2 Comprehensive genomic profiling liquid biopsy CDx platforms

Platform	Target genes/ biomarkers	Indication	Sample type	Technology	Regulatory status	Strengths	Limitations
FoundationOne Liquid CDx	324 genes, TMB, MSI, CNAs	All solid tumors	Plasma	Hybrid-capture NGS	FDA CDx (USA), CE-IVD (EU)	Broad profiling; approved for multiple therapies	VAF sensitivity varies by tumor
Guardant360 CDx	>70 genes	NSCLC, others	Plasma	Hybrid-capture NGS	FDA CDx (USA), CE-IVD (EU)	High concordance, fast mutation detection	Reduced sensitivity in low-shedding tumors
InVisionFirst-Lung	36 genes	NSCLC	Plasma	Hybrid-capture NGS	LDT (USA, CLIA) CE-IVD (EU)	Noninvasive, useful when tissue is unavailable	Not FDA CDx; lacks single-drug linkage
Archer Reveal ctDNA 28	28 genes	Solid tumors	Plasma	AMP-NGS + UMIs	RUO (USA) CE-IVD (limited EU)	High accuracy in plasma; quick results	Some findings may lack clinical actionability
MSK-ACCESS	129 genes	Solid tumors	Plasma + WBC	Duplex UMI NGS	NYSDOH certified (USA)	CHIP filtering; ultralow VAF detection	Not FDA approved; limited in MRD monitoring
OncoSTRAT&GO	192 (tissue) + 27 (plasma) genes	Metastatic solid tumors	FFPE + plasma	Ion AmpliSeq NGS	CE-IVD (EU); institutional use (global)	Reflects clonal evolution & heterogeneity	Discordance interpretation complexity
PGDx elio™ plasma resolve	33 genes + MSI	Solid tumors	Plasma	NGS	LDT (USA) CE-IVD (EU)	MSI detection in ctDNA; noninvasive profiling	MSI false negatives are possible
AVENIO ctDNA Targeted Kit	17 genes	Solid tumors	Plasma	NGS	RUO (USA) CE-IVD (EU)	Detects low VAF mutations; NCCN-based panel	Limited for ultralow VAF, early disease
QIAseq Targeted DNA Panel	Customizable panels	Solid tumors	Plasma	UMI-NGS	RUO (global)	Low DNA input; error-correction via UMIs	Not clinically validated for treatment decisions
Oncomine cfNA Assay	52 genes	Solid tumors, CNS	Plasma, CSF	NGS	RUO (USA) CE-IVD (EU)	CSF compatibility; high sensitivity	No FDA CDx; mostly for research use

high clinical responsiveness observed. Additionally, plasma NGS significantly reduced turnaround time (TAT) compared to tissue-based NGS (9 days vs. 20 days, $p < 0.001$), thereby expediting clinical decision-making. For key actionable mutations such as EGFR exon 19 deletion, L858R, and T790M, plasma testing demonstrated reliability comparable to that of tissue testing, and plasma-based mutation detection was directly associated with TKI responsiveness and progression-free survival (PFS) [5, 31]. In another study, Archer Reveal ctDNA™ 28 was rigorously validated through comparison with digital droplet PCR (ddPCR) [60]. Through ultra-deep sequencing, a high sensitivity (96%) and specificity (100%) were observed even at a variant allele frequency (VAF) of 0.5% [38, 62]. However, sensitivity decreased somewhat at ultralow variant concentrations below 0.1% [62, 63]. This suggests that ddPCR may have a relative advantage in detecting ultralow-frequency variants. The concordance rate for variant detection between the two methods was 91%, and it was confirmed to be particularly effective for monitoring treatment response in NSCLC patients receiving TKI therapy. These results indicate that while the detection limit of Archer Reveal ctDNA™ 28 may be somewhat restricted compared to ddPCR, it offers clear advantages in simultaneous multigene analysis and in expanding the range of detectable actionable mutations. In summary, Archer Reveal ctDNA™ 28 is a blood-based, noninvasive platform that enables rapid and accurate molecular profiling of solid tumor patients. It can be flexibly applied in various clinical scenarios, including treatment response monitoring, detection of resistance mutations, and early relapse detection, playing a crucial role in the implementation of precision medicine. However, the 28-gene panel includes variants that are not clinically actionable, so results may not always translate directly into therapeutic strategies. In practice, if no driver mutation is detected or if a mutation is identified but no appropriate targeted therapy is available, clinical utility is limited. To date, validation has primarily focused on NSCLC, but large-scale prospective clinical validation is needed for other solid tumors such as gastric, colorectal, pancreatic, and breast cancers. If further evidence is accumulated through multicenter, multi-cancer studies, Archer Reveal ctDNA™ 28 has significant potential to become a key tool for precision medicine across various cancer types.

5.3.5 Inivata InVisionFirst-Lung

Although tissue biopsy remains the standard for molecular diagnosis in non-small cell lung cancer (NSCLC) patients, in real-world clinical practice, issues such as insufficient tissue quantity, risks associated with invasive procedures, and difficulty accessing metastatic lesions are frequently encountered. These limitations often delay or preclude the acquisition of molecular information necessary for treatment decisions, thereby restricting therapeutic opportunities for patients. To address these clinical challenges, Inivata developed InVisionFirst-Lung, a blood-based liquid biopsy platform that analyzes circulating tumor DNA (ctDNA) in plasma to detect mutations in 36 cancer-related genes [64]. This system utilizes Inivata's proprietary Enhanced Tagged-Amplicon Sequencing (eTAm-Seq™) technology and is optimized for the detection of ultralow frequency variants, thereby positioning this platform as an alternative or complementary approach to conventional tissue-based analysis. The clinical performance of this assay was first systematically validated in a prospective multicenter clinical trial (INI-001, NCT0290652) reported in 2019. A total of 264 treatment-naïve patients with advanced NSCLC were enrolled; of these, 178 were included in the analysis group for direct comparison with tissue-based genomic analysis, while 86 were classified as patients with inadequate or unavailable tissue samples. The study found a concordance rate of 97.8% for mutation detection between InVisionFirst-Lung and tissue-based testing. For the eight key genes critical to treatment decisions (including EGFR, ALK, ROS1, and BRAF), the assay demonstrated a sensitivity of 73.9%, specificity of 99.8%, positive predictive value of 97.8%, and negative predictive value of 97.1%. This indicates that plasma-based testing provides a level of reliability nearly equivalent to tissue-based analysis. Furthermore, in the patient group without available tissue samples, InVisionFirst-Lung identified new actionable mutations, thereby identifying approximately 26% more patients eligible for targeted therapy, including those not detected by tissue testing alone. These findings demonstrate that this assay is not merely an alternative but can actually expand therapeutic options for real-world patient populations. Subsequently, the GRN-ALV study (NCT03116633) reported in 2022 evaluated the performance of InVisionFirst-Lung in a larger patient cohort [29]. A total of 803 patients with advanced NSCLC were included, and across the study, the concordance rate for variant detection between tissue-based and plasma-based assays remained above 97%. Notably, actionable mutations were identified in approximately 35% of all patients, and EGFR mutation detection was strongly associated with TKI treatment response and progression-free survival (PFS). Additionally, the turnaround time (TAT) for reporting results was significantly shorter for plasma-based assays, averaging 7–10 days, compared to an average of 20 days for tissue-based analysis, thereby enabling more rapid clinical decision-making. This is of significant clinical value in the management of patients with advanced lung cancer, where prompt initiation of therapy is directly linked to prognosis.

InVisionFirst-Lung is also expanding its research scope to include recurrence monitoring and minimal residual disease (MRD) detection. In the NCT04153526 study, a total of 363 serial plasma samples were collected from 88 patients with early-stage (NSCLC stage I–III) disease for ctDNA analysis. The preoperative ctDNA detection rates were reported as 24% in stage I, 77% in stage II, and 87% in stage III patients. The median tumor fraction of detected ctDNA was only 0.042%, with 63% of all samples at or below 0.1%, and a substantial proportion below 0.01%, indicating ultralow concentrations. Nevertheless, ctDNA analysis maintained a specificity of over 98.5%, and the time point of ctDNA detection in relapsed patients preceded clinical recurrence diagnosis by an average of 212.5 days (approximately 7 months). Among 28 patients who experienced recurrence, ctDNA was detected in 18 (64.3%), and in 17% of all cases, ctDNA was identified between 2 weeks and 4 months after completion of therapy. These patients exhibited poor relapse-free survival (RFS, HR = 14.8, $p < 0.00001$) and overall survival (OS, HR = 5.48, $p < 0.0003$). These findings support the substantial clinical utility of InVisionFirst-Lung for MRD detection and early prediction of recurrence.

However, InVisionFirst-Lung has not yet received official FDA approval as a Companion Diagnostic (CDx). This is interpreted not as a result of technical limitations, but ratheras reflecting differences in regulatory and commercial strategies. Approval as a Companion Diagnostic requires strong co-development with a specific drug. For example, the cobas® EGFR Mutation Test v2 was approved in direct association with osimertinib (TAGRISSO®), and the therascreen® PIK3CA RGQ PCR Kit with alpelisib (PIQRAY®).

In contrast, InVisionFirst-Lung was designed as a comprehensive genomic profiling (CGP) platform to support the selection of various targeted therapies, rather than being limited to a single drug, and did not pursue a co-development pathway with multinational pharmaceutical companies. Currently, the test is commercially available in the United States as a Laboratory Developed Test (LDT) through CLIA-certified laboratories and is widely used in clinical practice without the need for FDA approval.

In conclusion, InVisionFirst-Lung enables the detection of actionable mutations even in situations where tissue biopsy is difficult or limited and serves as a precision diagnostic platform encompassing target selection for therapy, detection of resistance mutations, MRD assessment, and early prediction of recurrence. Its high concordance and clinical validity have already been demonstrated in multicenter prospective clinical studies, and there remains significant potential for future expansion of CDx indications through linkage with specific drugs.

5.3.6 MSK-ACCESS

MSK-ACCESS (Memorial Sloan Kettering–Analysis of Circulating cfDNA to Examine Somatic Status) is a liquid biopsy platform developed for the high-precision detection of somatic mutations in ultralow concentrations of circulating tumor DNA (ctDNA) [49]. This assay targets a total of 129 cancer-related genes and comprehensively detects various genetic alterations, including single-nucleotide variants (SNVs), insertions/deletions (indels), copy number alterations, and fusions/rearrangements. The panel design is based on over 25,000 solid tumor genomic datasets from the tissue-based MSK-IMPACT panel clinically used at Memorial Sloan Kettering Cancer Center, with target genes selected for their direct association with FDA-approved drugs or their status as actionable biomarkers in clinical trials. As a result, MSK-ACCESS was designed to cover a total of 826 exons and 40 intronic regions, including rearrangement hotspot areas. Technically, by introducing a unique molecular index (UMI), sequencing errors are eliminated, and high accuracy is maintained even for ultralow-frequency variants through the generation of duplex consensus reads.

Initial clinical validation of the platform was conducted using 681 blood samples collected from a total of 617 cancer patients. Analysis revealed that cfDNA variants were detected in 73% of all cases. Among these, 56% were classified as clinically actionable mutations, and according to OncoKB criteria, 41% fell within Level 1–3B, indicating immediate applicability for FDA-approved therapies or clinical trials. Variant allele frequency (VAF) could be detected down to 0.02%, and even at VAFs below 0.5%, sensitivity was reported at 92% and specificity at over 99%. Notably, when compared with tissue-based MSK-IMPACT, the overall concordance rate for variant detection was 59%, with 20% detected only in blood-based (MSK-ACCESS) and 21% only in tissue-based assays. Of the variants detected exclusively in blood, 12% were evaluated as actionable mutations, demonstrating that MSK-ACCESS can complement tissue biopsy and expand therapeutic opportunities.

False positives, a common issue in liquid biopsy, mainly arise from clonal hematopoiesis (CH) or germline mutations [65]. To address this, MSK-ACCESS employs a strategy of parallel sequencing of white blood cell (WBC) DNA from the same patient to compare and filter cfDNA variants.

Subsequent analyses showed that this process eliminated over 10,000 variant events, the majority of which were CH-related variants that could have been reported as noise by commercial cfDNA platforms. This WBC filtering approach fundamentally enhances the precision of ctDNA analysis by minimizing the risk of unnecessary treatment due to false-positive signals in actual patient management.

The clinical utility of MSK-ACCESS was further demonstrated with real-world application data. In a cohort of patients with advanced solid tumors, plasma cfDNA analysis led to the identification of actionable mutations, which in turn guided therapeutic selection and clinical trial enrollment, resulting in tangible changes in patient management. Particularly, in cases where tissue samples were insufficient or inaccessible, MSK-ACCESS, similar to InVisionFirst-Lung, newly identified patients eligible for targeted therapy, highlighting its distinct advantages in clinical practice.

However, compared to tumor-informed bespoke panels (e.g., Signatera, RaDaR), MSK-ACCESS is limited in the number of detectable variants and thus may exhibit relatively lower sensitivity in ultralow-frequency ctDNA analyses such as minimal residual disease (MRD) detection. Despite these limitations, MSK-ACCESS received clinical approval from the New York State Department of Health in May 2019. Although it has not yet obtained official FDA CDx approval, it is actively used for cfDNA analysis in solid tumor patients at multiple hospitals across the United States, including New York.

MSK-ACCESS is designed around three core principles: detection of ultralow-frequency variants, elimination of false positives using WBC-based filtering, and identification of clinically actionable mutations. It has firmly established itself as a liquid biopsy platform that complements tissue-based analysis. In particular, its high sensitivity and specificity, false-positive elimination strategy, and real-world impact on clinical decision-making underscore MSK-ACCESS as a leading liquid biopsy technology contributing to the realization of precision medicine beyond research use.

5.3.7 OncoSTRAT&GO

The OncoSTRAT&GO™ platform is a precision diagnostic solution for solid tumor patients that integrates tissue-based genomic analysis with liquid biopsy-based ctDNA analysis [34]. This system analyzes DNA extracted from formalin-fixed paraffin-embedded (FFPE) tissue and ctDNA isolated from peripheral blood, covering 192 cancer-related genes in the former and 27 in the latter, to comprehensively characterize the tumor's entire genomic landscape.

The analysis utilizes Thermo Fisher's Oncomine Comprehensive Panel v2 and, based on Ion AmpliSeq technology, performs ultra-deep sequencing at an average depth of 1000–10,000×, enabling detection of allele frequencies of approximately 5% or higher in FFPE samples and as low as 0.1% in plasma, thus optimizing sensitivity for both sample types [48, 62].

A representative prospective study was conducted on a total of 351 patients with stage IV solid tumors (including various cancer types such as breast, colorectal, lung, ovarian, prostate cancers, and sarcomas). Paired tissue and blood samples were collected from the same patients; solid tissue samples were required to contain at least 10% tumor cells, and only blood specimens that were stably stored without hemolysis were included in the analysis.

The analysis revealed that discordant variants between tissue and blood were identified in 86% of patients, of which 97% were determined to be clinically significant. Notably, 42% of variants detected exclusively in blood were directly associated with sensitivity or resistance to already approved anticancer drugs—approximately 80% of which were targeted therapies—and 54% met eligibility criteria for molecularly targeted clinical trials. The most frequently identified actionable variants included TP53, KRAS, and PIK3CA, which served as useful biomarkers for predicting response to hormone or targeted therapies.

In addition to spatial heterogeneity, temporal factors were also identified as major variables. The longer the interval between tissue biopsy and liquid biopsy, the lower the proportion of shared variants, and the higher the frequency of variants detected only in ctDNA. This is interpreted as a result of clonal evolution and selection pressure during treatment rapidly altering the tumor mutational landscape. For example, tissue obtained at diagnosis may not reflect molecular changes after treatment, whereas real-time ctDNA analysis can dynamically capture the molecular status at the time of therapy.

This study empirically demonstrated that liquid biopsy can complement the limitations of single-tissue biopsy in capturing tumor heterogeneity. OncoSTRAT&GO™ not only serves as an alternative to tissue-based analysis but also provides significant clinical value as an integrated tissue–blood molecular diagnostic platform for establishing personalized treatment strategies. It is particularly valuable as a diagnostic tool in cases where tissue biopsy is not feasible, repeated biopsies are limited, or the tumor molecular landscape changes rapidly during treatment, especially in patients with metastatic solid tumors.

5.3.8 PGDx elio Plasma Resolve

PGDx elio™ plasma resolve is an NGS-based liquid biopsy platform designed to precisely analyze plasma-derived circulating tumor DNA (ctDNA), enabling simultaneous detection of clinically significant genetic alterations and microsatellite instability (MSI) [14, 17]. Traditional MSI assessment has relied primarily on PCR or immunohistochemistry (IHC) using tumor tissue, but these methods are structurally limited when tissue sampling is not possible or specimens are depleted. Elio™ plasma resolve is one of the first commercial platforms capable of determining

MSI-H status using blood-based ctDNA, offering a clinical alternative that complements tissue-based diagnostics.

This platform comprehensively detects various types of alterations—including single nucleotide variants (SNVs), insertions and deletions (indels), copy number alterations, fusions, and MSI—across 33 key cancer-related genes. Leveraging advanced error correction algorithms and unique molecular identifiers (UMIs), it can reliably detect ultralow-frequency variants with a variant allele frequency (VAF) of 0.1% or higher in ctDNA.

In clinical validation studies, elio™ plasma resolve was used to compare tissue and plasma samples from 75 patients with solid tumors (both primary and metastatic). The concordance rate for variant detection was 77% in metastatic patients and 45% in primary tumor patients, indicating that ctDNA is more sensitively detected in metastatic disease. Concordance for MSI status was 87% overall, and some patients identified as MSI-H in plasma subsequently responded to immunotherapy, supporting the clinical validity of liquid biopsy-based MSI assessment.

Among the variants detected, the most frequently identified were TP53, KRAS, EGFR, PIK3CA, and, in some patients, FGFR2 amplification that was not identified by tissue-based testing was detected in plasma and subsequently confirmed by ddPCR validation. This case clearly demonstrates that ctDNA-based analysis can complement tissue testing by capturing mutations reflecting tumor heterogeneity and temporal evolution that may be missed by tissue biopsy. Additionally, elio™ plasma resolve, developed as a decentralized NGS platform, can be implemented at the hospital level, suggesting the potential for future adoption of distributed precision diagnostics [66]. PGDx elio™ plasma resolve is establishing itself as a precision diagnostic tool that overcomes the limitations of tissue biopsy and supports the development of personalized treatment strategies by simultaneously providing blood-based MSI-H detection and comprehensive mutation profiling. However, there have been reports of cases where MSI-H was not detected in plasma, indicating the need for further technological advancements to improve ultrasensitive detection. Nevertheless, this platform is supported by Q1-level studies that have demonstrated its clinical validity and reproducibility, and it is expected to be widely applicable in various clinical scenarios, including assessment of immunotherapy suitability and treatment monitoring. While PGDx elio™ plasma resolve has demonstrated the feasibility of ctDNA-based liquid biopsy, including MSI-H analysis, other platforms from the same company are designed to meet different clinical needs and research objectives. PGDx elio™ plasma complete is a comprehensive genomic profiling (CGP) panel targeting over 500 cancer-related genes, enabling simultaneous assessment of SNVs, indels, copy number alterations (CNAs), fusions, MSI, and plasma-based TMB (bTMB). This platform employs ultra-deep sequencing and error correction algorithms to enable precise molecular diagnostics even in patient populations with limited tissue accessibility. In particular, plasma complete provides researchers with extensive genomic information, facilitating the exploration of the clinical significance of variants not yet defined in clinical practice and supporting the discovery of new therapeutic targets. In contrast, PGDx elio™ plasma focus is a panel that selects 33 key genes to reduce turnaround time and enhance interpretive clarity. It includes actionable driver mutations such as EGFR, KRAS, BRAF, PIK3CA, ALK, and ROS1, which are directly relevant to therapeutic decision-making, and enables detection of mutations at low allele frequencies down to 0.1% through ultra-deep sequencing. Plasma focus is considered particularly suitable for rapid patient stratification and treatment planning in clinical settings. Among these, PGDx elio™ plasma focus Dx received De Novo approval (DEN230046) from the FDA in 2024, establishing itself as one of the officially approved liquid biopsy-based companion diagnostic (CDx) platforms. This assay enables broad detection of actionable mutations, including SNVs, indels, CNVs, and gene fusions, and the results can be directly used to determine eligibility for specific targeted therapies. Notably, as a decentralized NGS platform, it allows individual hospitals to perform testing independently, which is significant for improving diagnostic accessibility. In summary, the PGDx elio™ series forms a tiered portfolio addressing diverse clinical and research needs: plasma resolve demonstrates the clinical feasibility of MSI and ctDNA mutation detection, plasma complete supports research-driven comprehensive genomic exploration, plasma focus enables rapid detection of clinically critical mutations, and plasma focus Dx secures regulatory approval as a formal companion diagnostic.

5.3.9 Oncomine Cell-Free Nucleic Acid Assay

Oncomine™ Cell-Free Nucleic Acid Assay is a multiplex gene panel-based liquid biopsy platform designed for research use (RUO), enabling simultaneous analysis of cfDNA and cfRNA in plasma. This panel covers a total of 52 cancer-related genes and allows for the concurrent detection of various genetic alterations—including single-nucleotide variants (SNVs), insertions/deletions (indels), copy number variations, and gene fusions—in a single reaction. In particular, it demonstrates sensitivity capable of detecting variant allele frequencies (VAFs) as low as 0.1%, making it suitable for applications such as early cancer diagnosis, resistance monitoring during treatment, and recurrence surveillance, where detection of ultralow levels of ctDNA mutations is required.

Using the Oncomine cfDNA Assay, a comparative analysis of cfDNA from healthy individuals and cancer patients defined the normal cfDNA background pattern in liquid biopsy. This study highlighted that mutations observed in liquid biopsy are not necessarily cancer-specific and that distinguishing true from false mutations is critically important in high-sensitivity cfDNA analysis. The research contributed to establishing a normal reference range, enabling the Oncomine platform to provide not only mutation detection but also clinically reliable interpretation.

Additionally, the Oncomine cfDNA Assay has been applied to analyze ctDNA in the cerebrospinal fluid (CSF) of patients with central nervous system (CNS) tumors. In cases where tumor tissue is difficult to access or surgically obtained tissue is limited, cfDNA analysis in CSF enabled the detection of actionable mutations not identified in conventional tissue testing, demonstrating that liquid biopsy can serve as an alternative diagnostic tool for CNS lesions.

Furthermore, multiple independent studies have shown that the Oncomine cfDNA Assay provides high reliability in detecting key target mutations such as EGFR, KRAS, ALK, and BRAF, and can contribute to reducing the time required for clinical decision-making. In fact, the concordance rate between blood-based NGS testing and tissue-based testing has been reported in some studies to exceed 90%, with particular emphasis on the ability to detect additional actionable mutations in patient groups where tissue acquisition is not possible or is limited.

However, there are limitations. As a research-use-only (RUO) platform, it has not yet been approved as an FDA-authorized companion diagnostic (CDx), and thus, careful, investigator-driven interpretation and clinical application are required. Additionally, the 52-gene panel includes variants that are not clinically actionable, so detected mutations may not directly lead to changes in treatment strategy, and this should be taken into consideration.

Nevertheless, the Oncomine cfDNA Assay demonstrates significant potential for precision diagnostics based on liquid biopsy, owing to its ability to detect ultralow frequency mutations, comprehensive mutation detection from SNVs to fusions, and multilayered analysis including cfRNA. In particular, the establishment of normal reference patterns, application to CSF-based analysis, and clinical expansion across various cancer types are regarded as key evidence supporting the research value and clinical potential of this platform.

5.3.10 AVENIO ctDNA Targeted Kit

The AVENIO ctDNA Targeted Kit is an NGS-based liquid biopsy platform developed by Roche Sequencing Solutions, designed to precisely characterize the molecular landscape of tumors in solid cancer patients using circulating tumor DNA (ctDNA) from plasma [63]. This kit enables comprehensive detection of major tumor-related genetic alterations, including single-nucleotide variants (SNVs), insertions and deletions (indels), and copy number alterations (CNAs). It specifically targets 17 key cancer-related genes with high clinical utility, as emphasized in the NCCN guidelines. Representative genes include EGFR, KRAS, BRAF, PIK3CA, ERBB2, ALK, and ROS1, among others, and the kit can be directly linked to the selection of targeted therapies and assessment of treatment resistance in the management of various solid tumors, including NSCLC.

The analytical performance of the AVENIO ctDNA Targeted Kit has been systematically evaluated. Using reference plasma and serial dilution samples, the platform achieved 100% sensitivity for SNV detection at variant allele frequencies (VAFs) of 0.5% or higher. Furthermore, it was confirmed that detection of ultralow frequency mutations at the 0.1% VAF level is possible with approximately 50% sensitivity, even with an input of 20–40 ng cfDNA per sample. This performance is useful for detecting ctDNA in patients with extremely low tumor burden or early-stage cancer, and demonstrates the clinical potential of the system as an ultrasensitive liquid biopsy platform, supporting this conclusion.

In addition, the AVENIO ctDNA Targeted Kit has demonstrated high performance in terms of analytical reproducibility and data refinement algorithms. It showed consistent results in both intra-assay and inter-assay variability assessments, and the error suppression strategy to minimize false positive rates was effectively implemented. Notably, the ability to simultaneously detect indels and copy number variations, in addition to SNV detection, offers greater analytical flexibility compared to conventional ddPCR-based single mutation assays.

Clinically, the direct detection of actionable mutations such as EGFR T790M, KRAS G12C, and BRAF V600E in plasma provides significant value, particularly for patients in whom tissue samples are unavailable or limited, supporting therapeutic decision-making. Furthermore, dynamic monitoring of ctDNA concentration changes during patient follow-up can be utilized for treatment response assessment and early detection of recurrence.

In conclusion, the AVENIO ctDNA Targeted Kit, with its high sensitivity for mutation detection, multi-gene panel design, and robust performance even with low DNA input, can be regarded as a research-use-only (RUO) liquid biopsy platform with the potential to support clinical decision-making in early-stage cancer or low-tumor-burden patients, pending further validation. However, it is currently limited to research use only (RUO) and has not yet received official FDA approval as a companion diagnostic (CDx). Nevertheless, this platform is considered one of the key candidate technologies for ctDNA-based precision medicine, and further validation through large-scale prospective clinical trials is anticipated.

5.3.11 QIAseq Targeted DNA Panel

The QIAseq Targeted DNA Panel is a multiplexed NGS-based gene analysis platform developed by QIAGEN, designed to overcome structural limitations of conventional NGS analysis such as PCR duplicates, sequencing errors, and library bias by utilizing Unique Molecular Indices (UMIs). The UMI attached to each DNA fragment enables tracking of individual molecules, achieving digital-level mutation detection accuracy based on error correction, and providing highly reliable results even at low variant allele frequencies (VAFs).

The most significant technical advantage of the QIAseq system is its ability to reliably detect mutations with minimal input DNA (2–10 ng) [67]. This is particularly advantageous in clinical scenarios where plasma-derived cfDNA is limited, especially in liquid biopsy-based precision oncology. In fact, it analyzed 164 ancestry informative markers (AIMs) using the QIAseq Targeted DNA Panel and reported high reproducibility and accuracy even with low input DNA amounts. This study demonstrated the suitability of QIAseq technology for ultralow concentration blood-based sample analysis and demonstrated its feasibility for expanded clinical applicability.

Additionally, the QIAseq panel features a modular design, allowing users to customize specific gene sets according to research objectives or tumor types (customized panel design). This differentiates it from conventional NGS platforms that offer fixed single panels, making it suitable for cancer type-specific biomarker research, development of customized companion diagnostics (CDx), and multi-biomarker-based precision medicine.

However, while multigene assay platforms like QIAseq enable broad cancer genotyping, the direct correlation with improved clinical outcomes remains an active area of research. In particular, in ultralow VAF regions below 1%, background noise can complicate result interpretation, necessitating the development of additional correction algorithms and large-scale clinical validation. Therefore, the QIAseq Targeted DNA Panel is recognized for its strengths in precise analysis of ultralow concentration samples, customizable panel design, and error correction capabilities and is considered a technology with the potential to evolve from a research platform to a next-generation companion diagnostic platform.

5.3.12 FoundationOne Liquid CDx

FoundationOne® Liquid CDx is based on circulating tumor DNA (cfDNA) in plasma, a next-generation liquid biopsy test enabling comprehensive molecular profiling of solid tumor patients. It was the first comprehensive blood-based companion diagnostic (CDx) platform to receive approval from the U.S. Food and Drug Administration (FDA) in 2020 [46]. The test analyzes 324 cancer-related genes and is designed to detect single-nucleotide variants (SNVs), insertions and deletions (indels), copy number alterations, and gene rearrangements, as well as to assess tumor mutational burden (TMB), microsatellite instability (MSI), and tumor fraction.

The development of FoundationOne Liquid CDx was driven by the need to obtain precise molecular information in a less invasive manner, particularly for patient populations in whom tissue-based biopsies are challenging. Liquid biopsy has emerged as a practical alternative for patients with metastatic lesions confined to bone, or for those in whom tissue sampling is risky or likely to fail. Additionally, liquid biopsy can reflect multiple metastatic sites rather than a single lesion, offering the advantage of more accurately capturing tumor heterogeneity.

The core technology of FoundationOne Liquid CDx originated from Foundation ACT, which was initially launched for research use. Foundation ACT employed hybrid capture-based NGS technology to detect a variety of alterations—including single nucleotide substitutions, short insertions and deletions, gene rearrangements, and copy number alterations—across 62 target genes, even at low allele frequencies (AFs) [48]. This system utilized molecular barcode error correction to deliver highly reliable results from ultralow concentration cfDNA. Clinical performance evaluation reported an overall sensitivity of 99% (95% CI: 99.1–99.4%), with a sensitivity of 95% (95% CI: 94.2–95.7%) in the 0.25–0.5% VAF range. Building on this technological foundation and clinical experience, FoundationOne Liquid CDx expanded its analytical scope to 324 genes and evolved into a comprehensive genomic profiling (CGP) assay, incorporating MSI and blood-based TMB assessment.

FoundationOne Liquid CDx has demonstrated clinical validity and reliability through extensive validation studies involving more than 30 types of solid tumors. The platform's performance was evaluated using over 7500 samples and more than 30,000 unique variants. The detection limit for single-nucleotide substitutions and indels was set at 0.4% VAF and for gene rearrangements at 0.37% VAF. Copy number alterations could be detected when the tumor fraction was at least 21.7% (amplification) or 30.4% (deletion), and both MSI detection and blood-based TMB measurement were performed with high sensitivity. The false positive rate of the assay was extremely low at 0.013% (approximately 1 in 8000), and overall reproducibility was recorded at 99.59%. In accuracy analyses, comparison with conventional tissue-based results showed a positive percent agreement (PPA) of 96.3% and a negative percent agreement (NPA) of over 99.9% for single-nucleotide substitutions and indels [68]. These results establish FoundationOne Liquid CDx as a platform capable of reliably detecting a wide range of genomic alterations, including complex biomarkers such as MSI, bTMB, copy number alterations, and tumor fraction.

Clinically, FoundationOne Liquid CDx has been approved for multiple companion diagnostic indications. Notably, it detects EGFR activating mutations (Exon 19 Deletion, L858R) to assess eligibility for Osimertinib (TAGRISSO®) therapy and identifies PIK3CA mutations to determine suitability for Alpelisib (PIQRAY®) treatment [69]. It also evaluates BRCA1/2 mutation status to support treatment strategies with PARP inhibitors (such as Olaparib and Rucaparib), and confirms MSI-H status to guide indications for Pembrolizumab (Keytruda®) therapy.

Through this assay, actionable mutations have been identified in 65% of patients across more than 30 types of solid tumors, and in advanced prostate cancer, the detection of BRCA1/2 mutations and AR resistance mutations has been used to guide targeted therapy decisions [70]. In addition, in colorectal cancer patients, MSI-H status was accurately identified, enabling the distinction of patient groups eligible for immunotherapy [30].

FoundationOne Liquid CDx has established itself as a core tool in precision medicine by comprehensively reflecting the overall molecular landscape of tumors using only blood, thereby overcoming the limitations of tissue-based biopsies. In particular, it serves as an important alternative for patients in whom tissue sampling is impossible or limited, and it has the advantage of capturing tumor heterogeneity across multiple metastatic lesions.

However, there are still sensitivity limitations in ultralow concentration ctDNA with low VAF, and a negative result does not necessarily indicate the absence of mutations, highlighting the need to complementary use of tissue-based assays in clinical practice.

5.3.13 Guardant360 CDx

Guardant360® CDx is a representative comprehensive genomic profiling (CGP)-based liquid biopsy platform that utilizes circulating tumor DNA (ctDNA) in plasma. It is designed to provide a comprehensive molecular profile for patients with solid tumors. In August 2020, this assay received approval from the U.S. Food and Drug Administration (FDA) as the first blood-based NGS companion diagnostic (CDx) to guide the use of specific targeted therapies in patients with non-small cell lung cancer (NSCLC) [4].

At the time of approval, the primary indication was to assess eligibility for Osimertinib (TAGRISSO®) therapy by detecting EGFR exon 19 deletion, exon 21 L858R, and exon 20 T790M mutations [6]. As a result, Guardant360® CDx became a clinically reliable alternative for patients in whom tissue biopsy is difficult or insufficient and was established as the first FDA-approved blood-based NGS companion diagnostic. Subsequently, its CDx indication was expanded to include the detection of EGFR exon 20 insertion mutations to determine eligibility for Amivantamab (RYBREVANT™), thereby playing a significant role in therapeutic decision-making for NSCLC patients.

Guardant360® CDx interrogates 74 genes by design, with a reportable range of 55 genes for single-nucleotide variants (SNVs), insertions/deletions (indels), gene rearrangements, and copy number alterations using high-depth hybrid-capture sequencing [61, 69]. In addition, it employs Guardant Health's proprietary error suppression algorithm, enabling high sensitivity; at 30 ng input, LoDs for many variants are ~0.2–0.5% VAF (variant-dependent), with higher LoDs at lower input. This analytical performance provides clinical advantages, achieving high concordance with tissue genotyping for FDA-approved targets and enabling dynamic monitoring via serial sampling.

For NSCLC, the assay supports therapy selection by detecting EGFR Ex19del, L858R, and T790M (osimertinib) and EGFR exon 20 insertions (amivantamab). The CDx label has also been expanded to include KRAS G12C (sotorasib), ERBB2 activating mutations (fam-trastuzumab deruxtecan-nxki), and ESR1 missense mutations (elacestrant). Like tissue-based assays, it supports both pretreatment decision-making and companion diagnostic purposes.

Its clinical utility has been demonstrated in numerous studies, among which the NILE Study (NCT03615443) provides the most robust evidence supporting the clinical validity of Guardant360® CDx [4]. This study enrolled 307 treatment-naïve Stage IIIB/IV NSCLC patients and conducted parallel analyses using tissue-based NGS and Guardant360® CDx. Among the 282 patients included in the final analysis, tissue-based genetic testing identified actionable mutations in 60 patients (21.3%), whereas Guardant360® CDx detected them in 77 patients (27.3%), demonstrating a significantly higher detection rate for cfDNA-based liquid biopsy compared to tissue testing ($P < 0.0001$). This confirmed the non-inferiority of cfDNA testing compared with tissue genotyping, with the additional advantage of a shorter turnaround time (median 9 vs. 15 days).

Concordance for FDA-approved target genes (EGFR, ALK, ROS1, BRAF) was reported to be over 98.2%, and among 34 patients with confirmed EGFR or ALK mutations, cfDNA and tissue biopsy results were in perfect concordance, achieving a positive predictive value of 100%. Notably, when including patients who received negative or inconclusive results from tissue biopsy, the number of patients in whom actionable mutations were detected by cfDNA analysis increased from 60 to 89, representing a 48% increase in detection rate. This demonstrates that Guardant360® CDx not only serves as an alternative to tissue-based testing but also provides additional therapeutic opportunities for patients. Large-scale subsequent real-world studies have further confirmed its clinical applicability. In an analysis of data from 21,807 patients with advanced solid tumors, a significant proportion of these were linked to improved therapeutic response and prognosis through matched targeted therapies. Additionally, Guardant360® CDx enables dynamic monitoring, with repeated reports highlighting its potential to track treatment response, emergence of resistance, and recurrence signals in real time. Of course, there are limitations. In patients with brain metastases or tumors that release very low levels of ctDNA, sensitivity may be reduced, and the possibility of false positives cannot be excluded if non-tumor cfDNA signals, such as those from clonal hematopoiesis (CH), are present. Therefore, interpretation of Guardant360® CDx results still requires WBC-based correction or integration with complementary tissue testing. Nevertheless, Guardant360® CDx has established itself as a tool that overcomes the physical and anatomical limitations of tissue-based biopsy, owing to its noninvasiveness, rapid turnaround, and high concordance. It is recognized as a leading companion diagnostic platform that enables the clinical implementation of precision oncology, including personalized therapy selection, detection of resistance mutations, and recurrence monitoring, not only in NSCLC but also in a variety of solid tumors. It is important to note that plasma-based ctDNA analysis for companion diagnostics is limited by its analytical sensitivity, and a negative result does not necessarily indicate the absence of genetic alterations within the tumor. In other words, when a specific mutation is reported as "not detected," this may simply reflect technical or biological factors that place the mutation below the detection threshold, rather than confirming that the mutation is "not present." This is a critical consideration in therapeutic decision-making, and caution is warranted in excluding treatment indications based solely on cfDNA analysis results. In particular, the presence of ctDNA in the bloodstream is influenced by various biological factors. When the tumor is small, at an early stage, localized to specific sites, or characterized by limited vascular invasion and low rates of cell death, ctDNA release may be extremely limited. In particular, ctDNA release may be markedly reduced in CNS-predominant disease (blood–brain barrier), in tumors with low burden, or in indolent histologies with low cell turnover. Therefore, in such situations, the sensitivity of liquid biopsy is inherently limited, and, if feasible, tissue-based testing or rebiopsy should be considered. In a comparative study of the MSK-IMPACT and GRAIL panels, among 124 patients in whom at least one mutation was detected by tissue-based genomic profiling, 20 patients (16%) had no tumor-derived mutations detected by cfDNA profiling. This is because ctDNA levels are often low or undetectable in patients with low tumor burden, certain cancer origins, specific histologies, or low levels of proliferation, apoptosis, and/or vascularization. From a technical perspective, FoundationOne® Liquid CDx shows an LoD of ~0.40% VAF for short variants and ~0.37% for rearrangements, and additionally reports MSI and blood-based tumor mutational burden (bTMB). Guardant360® CDx has reported an LoD in the range of approximately 0.2–0.5% VAF depending on mutation type and sample input (with lower input increasing the LoD) and has established drug-specific CDx indications for EGFR activating mutations (Ex19del, L858R, T790M) and EGFR exon 20 insertions. Thus, detection thresholds vary by mutation type and testing conditions, and the risk of missed mutations increases in the ultralow VAF (≤0.1%) range.

Another structural limitation is clonal hematopoiesis (CHIP). Clonal hematopoiesis of indeterminate potential (CHIP) refers to expansions of hematopoietic clones carrying somatic mutations in leukemia-associated driver genes, frequently observed in elderly individuals without hematologic malignancy. Large-scale solid tumor cohort studies have shown that a significant proportion of plasma cfDNA mutations (approximately half of the mutations reported in cancer patients) may actually originate from clonal hematopoiesis in the bone marrow rather than from the tumor itself, suggesting that systematic filtering using paired WBC sequencing is essential. In particular, mutations in genes such as DNMT3A, TET2, ASXL1, and TP53 can derive from either tumor or CHIP, making matched WBC DNA analysis indispensable for discrimination. In prostate cancer and other malignancies, there have been repeated reports that analysis of cfDNA alone can lead to misinterpretation. The DDR genes such as BRCA2, ATM, and CHEK2 are particularly vulnerable to CHIP-related misclassification, leading to erroneous PARP inhibitor eligibility.

In studies using MSK-IMPACT or GRAIL high-intensity cfDNA panels, concurrent cfDNA–tissue–WBC analysis showed that a large proportion of plasma variants are CHIP-derived, emphasizing the necessity of concurrent WBC sequencing. Notably, in patients with non-hypermutated solid tumors, more than half of the genetic mutations detected in cfDNA were found to originate from age-related CHIP rather than the actual tumor. Similarly, in a study analyzing cfDNA and whole blood (WBC DNA) from 69 patients with advanced prostate cancer, CHIP mutations were identified in 19% of all patients, and notably, 10% harbored mutations in DNA repair genes (ATM, BRCA2, CHEK2) associated with PARP inhibitor therapy eligibility [71]. The incidence of CHIP increases with age (e.g., ~30% in individuals ≥80 years; population studies typically report ~10–20% in those >70).

In cases where tissue-based genetic analysis is not feasible and treatment decisions must rely solely on cfDNA-based companion diagnostics, especially when the variant allele frequency (VAF) is low, there is a high risk of misinterpreting CHIP-derived mutations as tumor-derived, which can lead to serious errors in treatment selection. Indeed, the possibility of misdiagnosis due to CHIP-derived mutations has been reported in older men with advanced prostate cancer, indicating that differential diagnosis for CHIP is essential in cfDNA-based companion diagnostics.

If CHIP-derived mutations are misinterpreted as tumor-derived, patients may be unnecessarily or inappropriately prescribed targeted therapies such as PARP inhibitors, which can negatively impact both patient safety and treatment efficacy. Therefore, the latest studies consistently recommend that cfDNA-based testing should, whenever feasible, be accompanied by paired WBC analysis (or, at a minimum, rigorous filtering of canonical CHIP genes) to exclude CHIP-derived variants. For example, mutations in TP53, DNMT3A, TET2, and ASXL1 may originate from either tumor or CHIP, making comparative analysis with whole blood DNA essential for accurate discrimination.

The potential for false positives due to CHIP is thus a major limiting factor that can reduce the specificity of cfDNA-based assays, providing a rationale for why ctDNA testing cannot fully replace tumor tissue-based analysis. Ultimately, cfDNA-based testing should be used in a complementary role alongside tumor tissue analysis, and integrated interpretation of both approaches is required for accurate treatment decisions. In summary, cfDNA alone carries a persistent risk of reduced specificity, and exclusion of CHIP through concurrent WBC analysis is the current consensus.

In plasma-based analysis, there is always a risk that true tumor mutation signals present at low concentrations may be masked by background noise and go undetected, or conversely, that non-tumor-derived mutations may be misinterpreted as true tumor mutations. Therefore, even if actionable mutations are not detected in liquid biopsy-based cfDNA analysis, it is advisable to always perform tissue-based analysis in parallel during the diagnostic or therapeutic decision-making process. When feasible, repeat biopsy should also be actively considered. Ultimately, cfDNA results must be integrated with clinical context, histopathology, and imaging to ensure accurate decision-making, and repeat biopsy should be considered whenever feasible.

Despite the clear limitations described above, cfDNA-based genetic analysis remains a key alternative for implementing precision medicine in patient populations where tissue-based biopsy is not feasible or is limited. In particular, unlike tissue biopsy, which reflects only a single time point of tissue information, cfDNA offers the advantage of more comprehensively capturing the dynamic molecular evolution and tumor heterogeneity of malignancies in real time.

In early high-intensity cfDNA studies with a Grail 508-gene panel, high concordance with tissue was shown, while tissue testing often failed due to insufficient quantity/quality; paired WBC sequencing was used to identify CHIP variants. The main reasons for failure of tissue analysis were identified as insufficient sample quantity, low tumor cell content, inadequate DNA yield, and poor DNA quality. These issues were particularly pronounced in cases where metastatic sites were not amenable to biopsy, patients refused biopsy, or there were medical contraindications. In the SAFIR01/UNICANCER clinical trial, tissue genomic analysis was excluded in approximately one-third of patients with metastatic cancer, suggesting that cfDNA analysis, with its high compliance in real-world clinical settings, can serve as an alternative to tissue analysis.

Additionally, cfDNA-based companion diagnostics offer advantages in terms of turnaround time. For example, the NILE study demonstrated that Guardant360 CDx, which detects EGFR mutations via cfDNA, enabled treatment decisions to be made earlier than tissue-based analysis. This rapidity provides a clinically significant benefit, especially for high-risk patients in whom delays in initiating therapy may adversely affect prognosis.

In summary, the current consensus regarding the clinical application of cfDNA-based genetic profiling for companion diagnostics can be outlined as follows.

First, in patients for whom tissue biopsy is not possible or is difficult to access, cfDNA analysis can be considered the primary tool for companion diagnostics. This is particularly relevant when invasive biopsy is contraindicated or metastatic lesions are located in sites unsuitable for biopsy, making cfDNA-based testing the most practical option in terms of patient compliance. In fact, FDA-approved cfDNA companion diagnostic assays—such as the cobas® EGFR Mutation Test v2 and Guardant360® CDx—have been developed for these clinical scenarios and are effectively applied to guide targeted therapy selection in NSCLC, with selected FDA-labeled indications in breast cancer (ESR1 mutations).

Second, if no actionable mutation is detected in cfDNA—if the cfDNA test does not identify any genetic alterations—tissue-based genetic profiling must be considered as a complementary approach. This situation may arise when the variant allele frequency (VAF) in cfDNA is extremely low or in tumors that biologically release insufficient ctDNA into the bloodstream (e.g., indolent cancer subtypes, CNS-limited disease). Therefore, a "negative" cfDNA result does not necessarily indicate the absence of actionable mutations, and tissue analysis should be performed to supplement the final diagnosis, which is the consistent view among experts.

Third, when both tissue biopsy and cfDNA analysis are feasible, cfDNA analysis can serve as an additional diagnostic tool that reflects tumor heterogeneity and real-time molecular evolution. Especially in patients with advanced or metastatic solid tumors where a significant time has elapsed since the initial tissue biopsy, cfDNA analysis can enable early detection of acquired mutations, resistance mechanisms, or new actionable biomarkers that were not identified in the original tissue sample. This provides critical information for expanding therapeutic options and developing combination therapy strategies, underscoring the complementary value of cfDNA.

Fourth, if a genetic alteration is detected in cfDNA but not in the corresponding tumor tissue of the same patient, there is currently no clear consensus regarding the interpretation and clinical application of such findings. These discrepancies are frequently observed in clinical practice, and potential causes include tumor heterogeneity, limitations of cfDNA analysis, differences in sensitivity and specificity, clonal hematopoiesis, and various other factors have been raised. To date, it is recommended that such cases be approached on a case-by-case basis under expert judgment, taking into consideration each patient's disease stage, tumor location, and treatment history. In conclusion, cfDNA-based companion diagnostics cannot fully replace tissue-based genomic analysis, but they offer clear clinical value in terms of real-time analysis, ease of repeated measurements, and patient compliance. This suggests that tissue-based analysis and cfDNA analysis are not mutually exclusive but rather function complementarily. Integrated interpretation with tissue analysis can contribute to the realization of precision medicine, and clinical utility is expected to expand further through future integration with paired WBC analysis, ultralow frequency variant detection technologies, and multi-omics-based integrated interpretation platforms. In particular, liquid biopsy is anticipated to become a key tool for accelerating the implementation of precision medicine, especially when considering recurrence/metastasis timing, the emergence of resistance mutations, and issues of patient compliance.

5.4 Detection of Resistance Mechanisms

With advances in precision medicine, cancer treatment strategies are increasingly evolving toward designing personalized therapies based on molecular-level diagnostic information obtained from the patient's tumor (Fig. 5.5). This approach goes beyond traditional therapies applied to patient groups, aiming instead to maximize therapeutic efficacy and minimize unnecessary toxicity by precisely reflecting the individual patient's tumor genome and molecular characteristics. Such personalized treatment strategies can be broadly categorized into three key objectives: companion diagnostics, minimal residual disease (MRD) monitoring, and detection of resistance mechanisms, as previously described.

Companion diagnostics function as predictive tools that detect specific biomarkers or genetic alterations in a patient's tumor prior to treatment, thereby determining the suitability of targeted therapies in advance. MRD monitoring is used to detect minimal levels of tumor signals remaining in the patient's blood after surgery or chemotherapy, enabling early assessment of recurrence risk, adjustment of treatment intensity, and determination of the optimal timing for early intervention. The focus of this section, detection of resistance mechanisms, plays a crucial role in real-time identification of molecular changes that occur during or after treatment, allowing for early recognition of the onset and molecular basis of resistance and subsequent modification of therapeutic strategies.

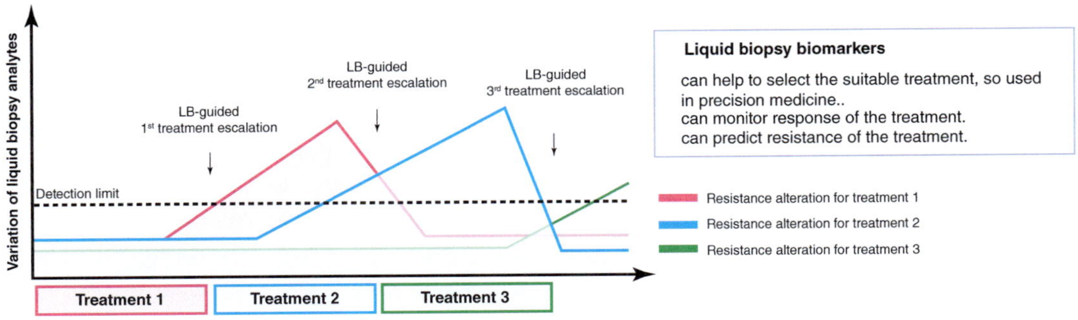

Fig. 5.5 Role of circulating biomarkers in treatment resistance

In particular, detection of resistance mechanisms involves capturing the molecular evolution of the tumor over time during the patient's disease course, which is distinctly different in clinical purpose and analytical strategy from companion diagnostics or MRD detection. In clinical practice, selection of targeted therapies still often relies on analysis of fixed tissue samples obtained at the time of diagnosis from the primary lesion. However, recent large-scale studies have demonstrated a high frequency of genetic discordance between primary and metastatic lesions, strongly suggesting that this is a result of treatment selection pressure and tumor evolution over time. Such heterogeneity is difficult to adequately capture through fixed tissue analysis alone, and especially at the time of metastasis or emergence of resistance during treatment, it is challenging to ensure both accuracy and timeliness of information—posing a significant limitation.

Tissue biopsy is not only invasive but also difficult to repeat, presenting inherent limitations. Furthermore, it does not comprehensively reflect intra-patient heterogeneity among metastatic lesions. The physical burden and risk of complications from repeated biopsies, consumption of medical resources, economic costs, and challenges in obtaining patient consent all pose significant constraints in actual clinical application. For example, in lung cancer patients, when performing repeated lung biopsies, the risk of pneumothorax can reach 15–20%, and in the case of liver biopsy, complications such as bleeding and infection have been reported. These practical limitations clearly demonstrate the need for new alternative technologies. On the other hand, liquid biopsy based on blood samples offers a unique advantage by enabling comprehensive analysis of cfDNA or CTCs released from various metastatic lesions, thereby reconstructing the overall tumoral molecular landscape. In particular, ctDNA serves as an analyte that allows for longitudinal tracking of tumor gene alterations over time, emerging as the most powerful tool for early detection of acquired resistance mutations that arise during or after treatment. Representative examples include EGFR T790M mutation (non-small cell lung cancer), ESR1 mutation (ER+ breast cancer), KRAS or BRAF mutations (colorectal cancer), and BRCA reversion mutations (PARP inhibitor resistance). Clinical evidence is accumulating that rapid detection of these mutations via liquid biopsy enables timely treatment modification, combination therapy, or enrollment in clinical trials. For the detection of therapeutic resistance, it is essential to go beyond simple identification of genetic mutations. One must also distinguish tumor-nonspecific mutations present in cfDNA, accurately interpret copy number alterations (CNAs), achieve ultrasensitive detection of low-frequency mutations, and exclude non-tumor mutations such as clonal hematopoiesis (CHIP). Failure to address these challenges may result in false positives or false negatives, potentially leading to inappropriate treatment decisions. In fact, in estrogen receptor-positive breast cancer patients, resistance mutations can accumulate years or even decades after diagnosis, leading to metastatic recurrence—an acquired molecular change that cannot be explained by initial tissue biopsy data alone [72]. In summary, while companion diagnostics focus on "pretreatment decision-making" and MRD monitoring contributes to "predicting posttreatment recurrence risk," the detection of resistance mechanisms enables "real-time monitoring of molecular changes during treatment." Thus, these three approaches, each with distinct temporal and analytical objectives, collectively serve as the three pillars of precision medicine encompassing the entire patient treatment journey.

Liquid biopsy is particularly well-suited for such longitudinal molecular tracking. Serial blood-based sampling can be performed repeatedly with minimal additional burden to the patient, allowing for early detection of treatment response and emergence of resistance mutations [44]. This enables proactive modification of existing therapeutic strategies and continuous optimization of personalized treatment. Recently, in various solid tumors, early detection of acquired mutations in key genes such as EGFR, ALK, ESR1, KRAS, BRAF, and BRCA via liquid biopsy has led to timely changes in therapy, application of next-generation inhibitors, introduction of combination regimens, or enrollment in clinical trials, with numerous cases reported. Accordingly, this chapter will focus on the roles that liquid biopsy can play in the detection of therapeutic resistance, centering on ctDNA and CTC analysis technologies. We will review in detail representative clinical studies and platform technologies conducted in metastatic solid tumors, types of molecular resistance mechanisms, and clinical application cases, and discuss in depth how liquid biopsy may contribute to the realization of precision medicine in the future.

There are two main strategies for detecting therapeutic resistance mechanisms using cfDNA-based analysis. One approach is exploratory, utilizing whole-genome or broad gene panels (>50 genes) to search for as-yet-unknown resistance mechanisms. The other is a targeted approach, which involves precise monitoring of already known specific gene mutations. The choice between these strategies depends on the analytical objective, tumor characteristics, and the patient's treatment stage, and both have complementary clinical significance. Whole exome sequencing (WES)-based cfDNA analysis is an exploratory strategy for identifying unknown resistance mechanisms. In cases where resistance pathways have not yet been clearly elucidated, WES-based cfDNA analysis can be a useful strategy for exploring mutations and clonal evolution that arise during treatment. Studies have reported the use of whole exome sequencing (WES) of serial plasma samples to investigate resistance mechanisms to chemotherapy or targeted therapies by tracking the genomic evolution of metastatic cancers. Six patients with advanced breast, ovarian, and lung cancers were followed for 1–2 years, with 2–5 plasma samples (a total of 19) collected and analyzed throughout the course of treatment. In a patient with HR+/HER2− metastatic progressive breast cancer, the mutant allele frequencies (MAFs) of PIK3CA, BMI1, and SMC4 increased after paclitaxel treatment; a truncated mutation in RB1 was identified after cisplatin therapy; and a truncated mutation in MED1 was detected following tamoxifen and trastuzumab treatment. In addition, various genes showed differences in MAFs before and after treatment depending on therapeutic response. However, WES of plasma cfDNA was only feasible in patients with a high proportion of ctDNA (≥5–10%). These findings suggest that cfDNA provides a means to monitor treatment-induced clonal evolution and acquired resistance mechanisms in real time, which cannot be detected by conventional tissue biopsy. Nevertheless, this approach is technically limited to patients with sufficiently high ctDNA fractions (≥5–10%), and the cost of analysis and complexity of data interpretation must also be considered. In contrast, for therapies with already known resistance mutations, targeted gene-based cfDNA analysis is more efficient and has greater clinical applicability. The targeted approach involves analyzing known resistance variants using a targeted panel or ddPCR-based methods. Highly targeted cfDNA analysis using genes associated with resistance to specific targeted therapies can provide strong evidence for validating preclinical hypotheses. For example, in the phase III clinical trial (PALOMA-3) of the CDK4/6 inhibitor palbociclib, a targeted panel (RB1, CDK4, CDK6, CDKN1A, CDKN2B, NF1, TP53, PIK3CA,

ESR1, ERBB2, FGFR1, FGFR2, FGFR3, AKT1, KRAS, NRAS, HRAS) was used to monitor tumor changes in 195 patients to elucidate mechanisms of resistance [72]. In the palbociclib plus fulvestrant group, RB1 mutations were detected in 6 of 127 patients (4.7%, $p = 0.041$), representing only a small subset of cases. Across both the combination and placebo groups, new mutations were identified during treatment in ESR1 Y537S ($p = 0.0037$) and PIK3CA ($p = 0.00069$).

The prevalence of RB1 mutations was found to be unexpectedly low among patients treated with CDK4/6 inhibitors. However, the ESR1 Y537S mutation promotes resistance to fulvestrant and leads to the emergence of driver mutations due to clonal evolution in later-stage patients, indicating distinct resistance mechanisms in both early and late phases of treatment. In colorectal cancer, cases involving anti-EGFR antibodies (cetuximab, panitumumab) clearly demonstrate that plasma ctDNA can provide early warning of resistance mutations before radiological recurrence [73, 74]. The monoclonal antibody cetuximab, which targets the epidermal growth factor receptor (EGFR), is known to be effective in patients with metastatic colorectal cancer (mCRC) who have wild-type RAS genes, particularly KRAS. However, this effect is mostly transient, and acquired resistance develops in many patients during treatment, limiting clinical benefit—a significant drawback.

One study analyzing metastatic lesions from mCRC patients who developed resistance to cetuximab or panitumumab reported that a substantial proportion exhibited acquired KRAS gene mutations. According to the study, secondary KRAS mutations were identified in the blood or tumor tissue of 60% (6/10) of patients who developed resistance, and KRAS gene amplification was also observed in one patient. These results provide strong molecular evidence that acquired alterations in the KRAS gene serve as a driving mechanism of resistance to anti-EGFR antibodies. Another study further demonstrated that this molecular evolution could be serially tracked. In patients receiving EGFR-targeted therapy, analysis of plasma ctDNA confirmed the emergence of KRAS mutant clones during or immediately after treatment. Notably, these KRAS mutant clones could be detected by liquid biopsy several months before radiological evidence of recurrence appeared, and in some patients, the mutant clones expanded rapidly within just 5–6 months after initiation of therapy. These studies provide two important implications. First, KRAS mutations act as key molecular events that induce acquired resistance to anti-EGFR antibody therapies such as cetuximab or panitumumab, indicating that tumor cells continue to undergo genetic selection and evolution even after the initiation of treatment. Second, cfDNA-based liquid biopsy can serve as a sensitive tool for early detection of these resistance mutations prior to radiological recurrence, offering opportunities for real-time therapeutic monitoring and timely adjustment of treatment strategies. Consequently, to address these molecular evolutionary pathways, early switching to subsequent therapeutic strategies such as MEK inhibitors at the time of KRAS mutation emergence in patients who initially responded to anti-EGFR therapy may provide clinical benefit. This approach could serve as a basis for developing real-time molecular monitoring algorithms to track treatment response and resistance. Osimertinib is a third-generation, selective EGFR-TKI designed to effectively target not only classical EGFR activating mutations (exon 19 deletion, L858R) but also the T790M point mutation (exon 20), a major mechanism of resistance. This agent has demonstrated superior clinical outcomes compared to standard chemotherapy (platinum plus pemetrexed) in T790M-positive non-small cell lung cancer (NSCLC) patients whose disease progressed after first- or second-generation EGFR-TKI therapy (e.g., gefitinib, erlotinib, afatinib). In the AURA3 trial, the efficacy of osimertinib was compared with platinum-based doublet chemotherapy (in combination with pemetrexed) in 419 patients with T790M-positive advanced NSCLC who had progressed after prior EGFR-TKI therapy. For the primary endpoint of progression-free survival, osimertinib achieved a median of 10.1 months, more than doubling the survival duration compared to 4.4 months in the chemotherapy group (HR = 0.30, 95% CI: 0.23–0.41, $p < 0.001$). Another notable finding from this study was the effect on patients with central nervous system metastases. Over 30% of all participants had brain metastases, and the osimertinib group demonstrated significantly superior objective response rates and progression-free survival in the CNS compared to chemotherapy. This result, together with the pharmacokinetic property of osimertinib to cross the blood-brain barrier, confirms its efficacy as a targeted agent capable of addressing systemic resistant mutant clones, including CNS lesions. Such clinical results strongly suggest that early detection and analysis of the T790M mutation can provide critical information for clinical decision-making. In other words, rapid determination of the T790M mutation status in patients with disease progression during EGFR-TKI therapy can serve as the starting point for selecting more precise treatment strategies beyond conventional chemotherapy. In particular, ctDNA analysis based on liquid biopsy can noninvasively and repeatedly monitor the dynamic emergence of T790M mutations even in patients with limited tissue accessibility, making it a key tool for determining the optimal timing for personalized treatment transitions. In cfDNA-based analysis of resistance mutations, broad panels such as whole exome sequencing (WES) are suitable strategies for exploratory research or early drug development stages where resistance mechanisms are not yet known, requiring relatively high ctDNA concentrations and sophisticated bioinformatics infrastructure for comprehensive variant detection and signal interpretation. In contrast, targeted analysis is advantageous when a clear causal relationship between a specific therapy and mutation has been established, and, relatively speaking, there are advantages in that results can be interpreted with high sensitivity and short analysis time even with low DNA input, making it more suitable for real-time application in clinical settings for monitoring therapeutic response and companion diagnostics. When considering future clinical applications, it will be necessary to establish guidelines for selecting cfDNA analysis strategies that comprehensively take into account the patient's cancer type, stage, treatment history, ctDNA concentration, and the purpose of analysis (exploratory vs. predictive). Whole exome sequencing (WES) and targeted analyses function as complementary tools and can be integrated as part of a flexible combination strategy for the implementation of precision medicine. In addition, copy number alteration (CNA) analysis is emerging as a notable strategy for detecting resistance mechanisms based on cfDNA. CNA refers to abnormalities in the copy number of specific genes or chromosomal regions and is closely associated with cancer development, progression, and therapeutic resistance. While tissue-based analyses allow for precise detection of CNAs, accurate detection has been challenging in liquid biopsy using cfDNA due to technical limitations.

In particular, most commercially available panel-based NGS platforms are optimized for detecting point mutations and indels, and therefore have limited ability to detect structural variants such as CNAs. However, with recent advances in broad sequencing platforms such as shallow whole genome sequencing (sWGS) and ultra-deep WGS, CNA analysis based on plasma cfDNA is becoming a reality. For example, in a study involving 127 patients with NSCLC, ultra-deep NGS analysis was used to detect resistance mutations in cfDNA. Among these, 17 patients were unable to undergo tissue biopsy, but cfDNA analysis alone successfully identified various acquired resistance mutations, including EGFR T790M (13 cases), EGFR C797S (1 case), ERBB2 amplification (2 cases), and KRAS mutations (4 cases). The variant allele frequency (VAF) of the detected mutations ranged from 0.14% to 52%, demonstrating that ctDNA analysis can serve as a practical tool to overcome the limitations of tissue-based testing. Additionally, a study utilizing shallow WGS to detect tumor-associated CNAs in cfDNA from prostate cancer patients demonstrated that large-scale genomic structural changes could be reliably detected in plasma, suggesting the potential to identify cancer type-specific CNA patterns. Similarly, an sWGS-based study in breast cancer patients detected FGFR1 amplification, which showed a significant correlation with reduced overall survival [75]. This indicates that CNA analysis can also serve as a prognostic biomarker. These studies provide two key insights. First, WGS based on cfDNA represents a technological advancement that can overcome the limitations of conventional gene panel-based NGS in detecting structural variants. Second, CNAs can serve as key biomarkers for predicting therapeutic response and prognosis, and the ability to quantitatively monitor them in cfDNA marks an important turning point in the assessment of metastatic disease and therapeutic resistance. Nevertheless, several technical challenges remain in cfDNA-based CNA analysis. Low cfDNA concentration, high background noise, and low tumor fraction negatively affect the sensitivity and accuracy of CNA detection. Shallow WGS, due to its low sequencing depth, has limitations in precision, and results may vary depending on the performance of interpretation algorithms. In summary, in cfDNA-based resistance analysis, WES/broad panels provide exploratory power in drug development or in cases of unknown mechanisms, while targeted analyses support rapid and highly sensitive clinical decision-making even at low concentrations. CNA analysis enables surveillance at the level of structural variants, broadening the scope of prognostic and therapeutic response prediction. In clinical practice, it is reasonable to design a customized hybrid strategy that integrates cancer type, stage, treatment history, ctDNA concentration, and the purpose of analysis (exploratory vs. predictive). For example, in the early stages, by using an expanded panel to explore candidate resistance pathways, and employing ddPCR or small panels in trackers for real-time monitoring of key mutations, a hierarchical algorithm that reassesses the genome-wide CNA landscape with sWGS upon signs of progression is clinically valuable.

It is well established that, in addition to circulating tumor cells (CTCs), associated cells and their products enter the bloodstream as cancer grows, evolves, and spreads. CTCs captured from a patient's blood respond sensitively to changes in the tumor microenvironment and therapeutic selective pressures, thus serving as a near real-time molecular and cellular snapshot of the patient's condition. In particular, the clinical value of CTCs in predicting prognosis and detecting mechanisms of therapeutic resistance in patients with metastatic cancer is increasingly recognized. For example, studies have shown that CTCs with ribosomal gene overexpression in patients with advanced metastatic cancer have been associated with poor prognosis, suggesting that CTCs themselves may serve as biomarkers for selecting therapeutic targets. This demonstrates that precise classification of CTCs based on phenotype and function, beyond mere presence or absence, can contribute to clinical decision-making. A representative example of CTC-based detection of therapeutic resistance is the identification of AR-V7 splice variant in patients with metastatic castration-resistant prostate cancer (mCRPC) [76–78]. AR-V7 (Androgen Receptor Splice Variant 7) is a ligand-independent, constitutively active androgen receptor known to be resistant to second-generation antiandrogens such as abiraterone and enzalutamide. The referenced study was the first to report that mCRPC patients with AR-V7-positive CTCs exhibited significantly increased resistance to abiraterone and enzalutamide, a finding that has since been repeatedly validated in subsequent studies. Further research has shown that the presence of AR-V7+ CTCs, defined by nuclear localization of AR-V7, is a reliable predictive biomarker for therapeutic response in castration-resistant prostate cancer.

Furthermore, the PROPHECY Study published in 2019 demonstrated in a multicenter prospective cohort that detection of AR-V7 at the mRNA or protein level could significantly predict progression-free survival (PFS) and overall survival (OS), independently of CTC count or established clinical prognostic factors [78]. This study suggests that the presence of AR-V7 is not merely a biological observation, but can function as a companion biomarker directly influencing therapeutic decision-making. In addition, CTC-based single-cell analysis is advantageous for elucidating molecular heterogeneity among various metastatic lesions within a patient, and, as a multi-omics platform capable of analyzing not only genetic information but also transcriptomic, proteomic, and functional characteristics, is expected to play a pivotal role in future research on therapeutic resistance. Another intriguing study sought to elucidate the genetic features associated with lung metastasis by using CTCs from patients with metastatic breast cancer in mouse model experiments. In this study, CTCs isolated from hormone receptor-positive (HR+) metastatic breast cancer patients were injected into immunodeficient mice, and CTCs recovered from metastatic sites showed markedly increased expression of genes encoding ribosomal proteins (RPs). Notably, CTCs with high RP gene expression also exhibited elevated expression of epithelial markers (such as EPCAM and CDH1), while expression of mesenchymal markers (such as VIM and FN1) was decreased, indicating an EMT-suppressed phenotype. These epithelial-rich, mesenchymal-low CTCs were closely associated with the induction of lung metastasis and were ultimately associated with reduced overall survival [79]. This study is regarded as an example demonstrating that, beyond mere detection, the transcriptomic and functional characteristics of CTCs can distinguish metastatic potential and prognosis. Although cfDNA/ctDNA can currently be measured more conveniently and in a more standardized manner than CTCs from a technical standpoint, CTCs provide unique biological information by directly capturing viable tumor cells. In fact, ctDNA is released through cell death or fragmented DNA released by necrosis can originate from various sources depending on the tumor microenvironment (TME), immune response, and metastatic sites. In contrast, circulating tumor cells (CTCs) reflect cells with metastatic potential that survive after treatment, making them a promising analyte for providing more direct information on metastatic potential prediction, therapeutic response analysis, and elucidation of resistance mechanisms. Notably, as platforms enabling single-cell level analysis of the genome, transcriptome, and proteome have expanded to include CTCs, there is a strong likelihood that CTCs will become established as a complementary precision diagnostic strategy alongside ctDNA. Nevertheless, the most widely used clinical indicator remains CTC enumeration, and the clinical value of CTCs as prognostic biomarkers has been validated in several advanced metastatic cancers, including breast, prostate, and colorectal cancers. Among 1944 patients with metastatic breast cancer, 911 (46.9%) had 5 or more CTCs per 7.5 ml of blood at the baseline timepoint, which was reported to be associated with reduced progression-free survival (PFS) [32, 37]. In addition, a sustained increase in CTC count at 3–5 weeks and 6–8 weeks after initiation of standard therapy was correlated with shorter PFS and overall survival (OS). While the clinical utility of independent prognostic assessment using CTC enumeration has been reported, conventional serum tumor markers used for posttreatment monitoring in breast cancer (CEA, CA15-3) did not improve prognostic accuracy. In prostate cancer, prognosis was assessed by enumerating CTCs in the blood of 37 patients after standard therapy and analyzing survival rates. The CTC threshold was set at 5; among the 37 patients, 23 (62%) had 5 or more CTCs, with a median overall survival of 0.7 years, whereas those with fewer than 5 CTCs had a median overall survival of 4 years, thus demonstrating the prognostic value of CTC enumeration in prostate cancer [38]. For colorectal cancer, the clinical utility of CTC enumeration as a prognostic cancer marker was confirmed in 430 patients with metastatic colorectal cancer [39]. Prognostic value was stratified based on a CTC threshold of 3. Patients with CTC counts below the threshold exhibited shorter PFS, thereby validating its prognostic significance. Another study involving 595 patients with metastatic breast cancer investigated both the prognostic value of CTC enumeration and therapeutic response. In this study, the effect of changing first-line chemotherapy on overall survival was evaluated in patients with persistently increasing CTC counts. Among patients who had received first-line chemotherapy for 21 days, those with persistently increasing CTC counts were divided into two groups: one continuing initial therapy and the other switching to alternative chemotherapy. Comparative analysis of survival rates showed no significant difference in median overall survival (10.7 months vs. 12.5 months, $P = 0.98$) [80]. These results demonstrate that while a sustained increase in CTC count may aid in prognostic assessment, it does not support the effectiveness of switching to alternative therapy based on CTC increase (therapeutic response).

To date, CTC enumeration has repeatedly demonstrated clinical utility as a prognostic indicator in various cancer types; however, its clinical usefulness as a predictor of therapeutic response has not been clearly established. In particular, as shown in the SWOG S0500 study, changes in CTC count did not lead to improved survival when directly linked to changes in treatment strategy, indicating that CTC enumeration has limitations as a decision-making indicator for therapy. This is largely due to the excessively low CTC thresholds set in most studies, which inherently limit both the sensitivity and specificity of the analysis when CTC counts are extremely low. Although correlations between posttreatment CTC counts and survival have been reported, there remain limitations in reliably predicting recurrence risk or drug responsiveness based on these findings. For example, when the threshold is set at 5 CTCs, the clinical interpretation of results between 4 and 6 CTCs can differ significantly, potentially leading to false-positive or false-negative assessments. The above studies utilized the CELLSEARCH system to capture and isolate CTC cell surface protein biomarkers. However, since CTCs collected in whole blood tubes are fixed, there are clear limitations to their use in drug sensitivity testing. As an EpCAM-dependent CTC analysis method, if it becomes possible to stably preserve living CTCs with cancer- or metastasis-specific surface protein biomarkers introduced or isolated from whole blood, the clinical utility of predicting therapeutic response could be improved. As a strategy to overcome these limitations, studies have been conducted on phenotypic and functional analysis of CTCs. Rather than simple enumeration, this approach aims to identify actionable targets and move closer to true precision medicine by directly assessing the molecular characteristics and drug responsiveness of viable CTCs. However, to date, clinical data supporting this approach remain limited, and technical and clinical validation is incomplete due to the rarity and heterogeneity of CTCs and the lack of standardized culture conditions. Nevertheless, several pioneering studies have demonstrated the potential of ex vivo models for evaluating anticancer drug sensitivity by culturing CTCs. A representative example is a study in which CTCs were isolated from the blood of small cell lung cancer (SCLC) patients, injected into immunodeficient mice to form tumors, and then used to assess drug sensitivity. Using the CELLSEARCH system, CTCs were isolated and injected into mice to establish patient-derived CTC xenograft (PDX) models, and responses to standard SCLC therapies such as platinum and etoposide were evaluated [35]. Consistent therapeutic responses were observed even in passage 4 PDx models, demonstrating the feasibility of CTC-based drug response assessment. In another study, CTCs were isolated and cultured from six patients with estrogen receptor (ER)-positive breast cancer to evaluate drug sensitivity [36]. After culturing CTCs obtained from patient blood ex vivo for several days, genomic sequencing identified not only preexisting PIK3CA mutations but also newly acquired ESR1 and FGFR2 mutations during treatment. This suggests that CTC analysis can enable real-time detection of treatment-induced clonal evolution and acquired resistance mutations. These studies demonstrate that, as viable cells present in small numbers in the bloodstream, CTCs can provide direct information on drug responsiveness that cannot be obtained from ctDNA-based analyses. In particular, as a tool for multidimensional analysis of the biological characteristics of cells with metastatic potential, CTC culture-based platforms are regarded as highly valuable strategies for implementing precision medicine. However, there are still significant limitations to clinical application. First, the extremely low abundance of CTCs in blood results in low experimental reproducibility. Second, culturing CTCs requires several days to weeks. Third, culture results may be available too late to inform clinical decision-making. Additionally, there is a lack of consensus on standardized culture conditions, drug panel composition, and criteria for interpreting responses. Therefore, further basic research and technical validation are needed for the clinical translation of functional analysis-based CTC companion diagnostic platforms, and it is now necessary to demonstrate their predictive validity for therapeutic response through longitudinal cohorts and prospective clinical study designs. When utilizing liquid biopsy to precisely detect mechanisms of therapeutic resistance, several key considerations must be kept in mind.

First, it is essential to understand the biological differences between analytes. ctDNA consists of fragmented DNA released by apoptosis or necrosis, which can sensitively reflect molecular alterations such as mutations and CNAs, but does not directly indicate the presence of cells with metastatic potential. In contrast, CTCs are viable metastatic cells that provide genomic, transcriptomic, proteomic, and functional information at the single-cell level and can inform on therapeutic responsiveness, which is advantageous for detecting the actual mechanisms of resistance. Since the two analytes are complementary, a combined analysis strategy is recommended to broaden the scope of interpretation.

Second, technical standardization and analytical sensitivity are crucial. Detecting ultralow-frequency ctDNA mutations or reliably isolating and preserving extremely rare CTCs requires highly sensitive and specific technological infrastructure. Tools such as UMI-based error suppression, duplex sequencing, EpCAM-independent capture methods, and single-cell analysis platforms are becoming essential, yet standardized procedures and international guidelines remain insufficient.

Third, exclusion of non-tumor signals is necessary. In ctDNA analysis, mutations such as DNMT3A, TET2, and ASXL1 originating from CHIP (clonal hematopoiesis of indeterminate potential) may be present, potentially leading to false positives. In CTC analysis, issues such as EpCAM-negative CTCs or nonspecific cell capture have also been noted. Therefore, sophisticated algorithms to filter out non-tumor signals are required for accurate interpretation.

Fourth, the sampling strategy is critical to the success of resistance detection. Systematic serial sampling should be implemented at baseline before treatment, during the early response phase (1–2 weeks), at the first imaging assessment (6–8 weeks), and at regular intervals thereafter (8–12 weeks). This design enables longitudinal tracking of molecular changes. If a dynamic risk score integrating VAF change rates, emergence of new clones, and clonal competition patterns is developed, it would allow rational adjustment of treatment strategies prior to radiological progression.

In summary, considering these factors, liquid biopsy is emerging as a core platform for real-time adjustment of patient-specific treatment strategies, surpassing its role as a mere adjunct in resistance detection. ctDNA sensitively tracks molecular changes to capture early signals of resistance, while CTCs provide complementary value by directly elucidating resistance mechanisms and drug responsiveness at the level of viable cells. Ultimately, integrated longitudinal monitoring of both analytes enables multidimensional capture of dynamic tumor evolution under therapeutic selective pressure and provides a foundation for precise adjustment of individual treatment trajectories. With the future development of standardized analytical methods, interpretive frameworks, and composite biomarkers, liquid biopsy could maximize its clinical impact as a key tool for resistance management and the realization of precision medicine.

References

1. Abbosh C, Birkbak NJ, Wilson GA, Jamal-Hanjani M, Constantin T, Salari R, et al. Phylogenetic ctDNA analysis depicts early-stage lung cancer evolution. Nature. 2017;545(7655):446–51.
2. Diehl F, Schmidt K, Choti MA, Romans K, Goodman S, Li M, et al. Circulating mutant DNA to assess tumor dynamics. Nat Med. 2008;14(9):985–90.
3. Merker JD, Oxnard GR, Compton C, Diehn M, Hurley P, Lazar AJ, et al. Circulating tumor DNA analysis in patients with cancer: American Society of Clinical Oncology and College of American Pathologists Joint Review. J Clin Oncol [Internet]. 2018 [cited 2025 Apr 29]; Available from: https://ascopubs.org/doi/10.1200/JCO.2017.76.8671
4. Leighl NB, Page RD, Raymond VM, Daniel DB, Divers SG, Reckamp KL, et al. Clinical utility of comprehensive cell-free DNA analysis to identify genomic biomarkers in patients with newly diagnosed metastatic non-small cell lung cancer. Clin Cancer Res. 2019;25(15):4691–700.
5. Aggarwal C, Thompson JC, Black TA, Katz SI, Fan R, Yee SS, et al. Clinical implications of plasma-based genotyping with the delivery of personalized therapy in metastatic non–small cell lung cancer. JAMA Oncol. 2019;5(2):173–80.
6. Mok TS, Wu YL, Ahn MJ, Garassino MC, Kim HR, Ramalingam SS, et al. Osimertinib or platinum–pemetrexed in EGFR T790M–positive lung cancer. N Engl J Med. 2017;376(7):629–40.
7. Cohen JD, Li L, Wang Y, Thoburn C, Afsari B, Danilova L, et al. Detection and localization of surgically resectable cancers with a multi-analyte blood test. Science. 2018;359(6378):926–30.

8. Schrag D, Beer TM, McDonnell CH, Nadauld L, Dilaveri CA, Reid R, et al. Blood-based tests for multicancer early detection (PATHFINDER): a prospective cohort study. Lancet. 2023;402(10409):1251–60.
9. Garcia-Murillas I, Chopra N, Comino-Méndez I, Beaney M, Tovey H, Cutts RJ, et al. Assessment of molecular relapse detection in early-stage breast cancer. JAMA Oncol. 2019;5(10):1473–8.
10. Coombes RC, Page K, Salari R, Hastings RK, Armstrong A, Ahmed S, et al. Personalized detection of circulating tumor DNA antedates breast cancer metastatic recurrence. Clin Cancer Res. 2019;25(14):4255–63.
11. Razavi P, Li BT, Brown DN, Jung B, Hubbell E, Shen R, et al. High-intensity sequencing reveals the sources of plasma circulating cell-free DNA variants. Nat Med. 2019;25(12):1928–37.
12. Shlush LI. Age-related clonal hematopoiesis. Blood. 2018;131(5):496–504.
13. Lennon AM, Buchanan AH, Kinde I, Warren A, Honushefsky A, Cohain AT, et al. Feasibility of blood testing combined with PET-CT to screen for cancer and guide intervention. Science. 2020;369(6499):eabb9601.
14. Shen SY, Singhania R, Fehringer G, Chakravarthy A, Roehrl MHA, Chadwick D, et al. Sensitive tumour detection and classification using plasma cell-free DNA methylomes. Nature. 2018;563(7732):579–83.
15. Chung DC, Gray DM, Singh H, Issaka RB, Raymond VM, Eagle C, et al. A cell-free DNA blood-based test for colorectal cancer screening. N Engl J Med. 2024;390(11):973–83.
16. Putcha G, Xu C, Shaukat A, Levin TR. Prevention of colorectal cancer through multiomics blood testing: the PREEMPT CRC study. J Clin Oncol 2022;40(4_suppl):TPS208.
17. Klein EA, Richards D, Cohn A, Tummala M, Lapham R, Cosgrove D, et al. Clinical validation of a targeted methylation-based multi-cancer early detection test using an independent validation set. Ann Oncol. 2021;32(9):1167–77.
18. Cristiano S, Leal A, Phallen J, Fiksel J, Adleff V, Bruhm DC, et al. Genome-wide cell-free DNA fragmentation in patients with cancer. Nature. 2019;570(7761):385–9.
19. Melo SA, Luecke LB, Kahlert C, Fernandez AF, Gammon ST, Kaye J, et al. Glypican-1 identifies cancer exosomes and detects early pancreatic cancer. Nature. 2015;523(7559):177–82.
20. Hoshino A, Kim HS, Bojmar L, Gyan KE, Cioffi M, Hernandez J, et al. Extracellular vesicle and particle biomarkers define multiple human cancers. Cell. 2020;182(4):1044–1061.e18.
21. Jeppesen DK, Fenix AM, Franklin JL, Higginbotham JN, Zhang Q, Zimmerman LJ, et al. Reassessment of exosome composition. Cell. 2019;177(2):428–445.e18.
22. Xenidis N, Ignatiadis M, Apostolaki S, Perraki M, Kalbakis K, Agelaki S, et al. Cytokeratin-19 mRNA-positive circulating tumor cells after adjuvant chemotherapy in patients with early breast cancer. J Clin Oncol Off J Am Soc Clin Oncol. 2009;27(13):2177–84.
23. Trapp E, Janni W, Schindlbeck C, Jückstock J, Andergassen U, de Gregorio A, et al. Presence of circulating tumor cells in high-risk early breast cancer during follow-up and prognosis. J Natl Cancer Inst. 2019;111(4):380–7.
24. Riethdorf S, Müller V, Loibl S, Nekljudova V, Weber K, Huober J, et al. Prognostic impact of circulating tumor cells for breast cancer patients treated in the Neoadjuvant "Geparquattro" trial. Clin Cancer Res. 2017;23(18):5384–93.
25. Best MG, Sol N, Kooi I, Tannous J, Westerman BA, Rustenburg F, et al. RNA-Seq of tumor-educated platelets enables blood-based pan-cancer, multiclass, and molecular pathway cancer diagnostics. Cancer Cell. 2015;28(5):666–76.
26. Tie J, Wang Y, Lo SN, Lahouel K, Cohen JD, Wong R, et al. Circulating tumor DNA analysis guiding adjuvant therapy in stage II colon cancer: 5-year outcomes of the randomized DYNAMIC trial. Nat Med. 2025;31:1509–18.
27. Kotani D, Oki E, Nakamura Y, Yukami H, Mishima S, Bando H, et al. Molecular residual disease and efficacy of adjuvant chemotherapy in patients with colorectal cancer. Nat Med. 2023;29(1):127–34.
28. McDonald BR, Contente-Cuomo T, Sammut SJ, Odenheimer-Bergman A, Ernst B, Perdigones N, et al. Personalized circulating tumor DNA analysis to detect residual disease after neoadjuvant therapy in breast cancer. Sci Transl Med. 2019;11(504):eaax7392.
29. Gale D, Heider K, Ruiz-Valdepenas A, Hackinger S, Perry M, Marsico G, et al. Residual ctDNA after treatment predicts early relapse in patients with early-stage non-small cell lung cancer. Ann Oncol. 2022;33(5):500–10.
30. Venook AP. Colorectal cancer surveillance with circulating tumor DNA assay. JAMA Netw Open. 2022;5(3):e221100.
31. Sabari JK, Offin M, Stephens D, Ni A, Lee A, Pavlakis N, et al. A prospective study of circulating tumor DNA to guide matched targeted therapy in lung cancers. J Natl Cancer Inst. 2019;111(6):575–83.
32. Cristofanilli M, Budd GT, Ellis MJ, Stopeck A, Matera J, Miller MC, et al. Circulating tumor cells, disease progression, and survival in metastatic breast cancer. N Engl J Med. 2004;351(8):781–91.
33. Schuster E, Taftaf R, Reduzzi C, Albert MK, Romero-Calvo I, Liu H. Better together: circulating tumor cell clustering in metastatic cancer. Trends Cancer. 2021;7(11):1020–32.
34. Finzel A, Sadik H, Ghitti G, Laes JF. The combined analysis of solid and liquid biopsies provides additional clinical information to improve patient care. J Cancer Metastasis Treat. 2018;4:21.
35. Yu M, Bardia A, Aceto N, Bersani F, Madden MW, Donaldson MC, et al. Ex vivo culture of circulating breast tumor cells for individualized testing of drug susceptibility. Science. 2014;345(6193):216–20.
36. Hodgkinson CL, Morrow CJ, Li Y, Metcalf RL, Rothwell DG, Trapani F, et al. Tumorigenicity and

genetic profiling of circulating tumor cells in small-cell lung cancer. Nat Med. 2014;20(8):897–903.
37. Hayes DF, Cristofanilli M, Budd GT, Ellis MJ, Stopeck A, Miller MC, et al. Circulating tumor cells at each follow-up time point during therapy of metastatic breast cancer patients predict progression-free and overall survival. Clin Cancer Res. 2006;12(14 Pt 1):4218–24.
38. Moreno JG, Miller MC, Gross S, Allard WJ, Gomella LG, Terstappen LWMM. Circulating tumor cells predict survival in patients with metastatic prostate cancer. Urology. 2005;65(4):713–8.
39. Cohen SJ, Punt CJA, Iannotti N, Saidman BH, Sabbath KD, Gabrail NY, et al. Prognostic significance of circulating tumor cells in patients with metastatic colorectal cancer. Ann Oncol Off J Eur Soc Med Oncol. 2009;20(7):1223–9.
40. Sparano J, O'Neill A, Alpaugh K, Wolff AC, Northfelt DW, Dang CT, et al. Association of circulating tumor cells with late recurrence of estrogen receptor-positive breast cancer: a secondary analysis of a randomized clinical trial. JAMA Oncol. 2018;4(12):1700–6.
41. Goodman CR, Seagle BLL, Friedl TWP, Rack B, Lato K, Fink V, et al. Association of circulating tumor cell status with benefit of radiotherapy and survival in early-stage breast cancer. JAMA Oncol. 2018;4(8):e180163.
42. Bidard FC, Jacot W, Kiavue N, Dureau S, Kadi A, Brain E, et al. Efficacy of circulating tumor cell count-driven vs clinician-driven first-line therapy choice in hormone receptor-positive, ERBB2-negative metastatic breast cancer: the STIC CTC randomized clinical trial. JAMA Oncol. 2021;7(1):34–41.
43. Bidard FC, Kiavue N, Jacot W, Bachelot T, Dureau S, Bourgeois H, et al. Overall survival with circulating tumor cell count–driven choice of therapy in advanced breast cancer: a randomized trial. J Clin Oncol [Internet] 2024 [cited 2025 Sep 2]; Available from: https://ascopubs.org/doi/10.1200/JCO.23.00456
44. Murtaza M, Dawson SJ, Tsui DWY, Gale D, Forshew T, Piskorz AM, et al. Non-invasive analysis of acquired resistance to cancer therapy by sequencing of plasma DNA. Nature. 2013;497(7447):108–12.
45. Heitzer E, Ulz P, Belic J, Gutschi S, Quehenberger F, Fischereder K, et al. Tumor-associated copy number changes in the circulation of patients with prostate cancer identified through whole-genome sequencing. Genome Med. 2013;5(4):30.
46. Woodhouse R, Li M, Hughes J, Delfosse D, Skoletsky J, Ma P, et al. Clinical and analytical validation of FoundationOne liquid CDx, a novel 324-gene cfDNA-based comprehensive genomic profiling assay for cancers of solid tumor origin. PLoS One. 2020;15(9):e0237802.
47. Gydush G, Nguyen E, Bae JH, Blewett T, Rhoades J, Reed SC, et al. Massively parallel enrichment of low-frequency alleles enables duplex sequencing at low depth. Nat Biomed Eng. 2022;6(3):257–66.
48. Clark TA, Chung JH, Kennedy M, Hughes JD, Chennagiri N, Lieber DS, et al. Analytical validation of a hybrid capture-based next-generation sequencing clinical assay for genomic profiling of cell-free circulating tumor DNA. J Mol Diagn JMD. 2018;20(5):686–702.
49. Rose Brannon A, Jayakumaran G, Diosdado M, Patel J, Razumova A, Hu Y, et al. Enhanced specificity of clinical high-sensitivity tumor mutation profiling in cell-free DNA via paired normal sequencing using MSK-ACCESS. Nat Commun. 2021;12(1):3770.
50. Bidard FC, Kiavue N, Ychou M, Cabel L, Stern MH, Madic J, et al. Circulating tumor cells and circulating tumor DNA detection in potentially resectable metastatic colorectal cancer: a prospective ancillary study to the Unicancer Prodige-14 trial. Cells. 2019;8(6):516.
51. Parsons HA, Blewett T, Chu X, Sridhar S, Santos K, Xiong K, et al. Circulating tumor DNA association with residual cancer burden after neoadjuvant chemotherapy in triple-negative breast cancer in TBCRC 030☆. Ann Oncol. 2023;34(10):899–906.
52. United States Food and Drug Administration. Premarket Approval (PMA) application P150047 [Internet]. Silver Spring (MD): FDA; 2015 [cited 2025 Sep 24]. Available from: https://www.accessdata.fda.gov/scripts/cdrh/cfdocs/cfpma/pma.cfm?id=P150047
53. United States Food and Drug Administration. Premarket Approval (PMA) application P190004 [Internet]. Silver Spring (MD): FDA; 2019 [cited 2025 Sep 24]. Available from: https://www.accessdata.fda.gov/scripts/cdrh/cfdocs/cfpma/pma.cfm?id=P190004
54. André F, Ciruelos E, Rubovszky G, Campone M, Loibl S, Rugo HS, et al. Alpelisib for PIK3CA-mutated, hormone receptor-positive advanced breast cancer. N Engl J Med. 2019;380(20):1929–40.
55. André F, Ciruelos EM, Juric D, Loibl S, Campone M, Mayer IA, et al. Alpelisib plus fulvestrant for PIK3CA-mutated, hormone receptor-positive, human epidermal growth factor receptor-2-negative advanced breast cancer: final overall survival results from SOLAR-1. Ann Oncol Off J Eur Soc Med Oncol. 2021;32(2):208–17.
56. United States Food and Drug Administration. Premarket Approval (PMA) application P210040 [Internet]. Silver Spring (MD): FDA; 2021 [cited 2025 Sep 24]. Available from: https://www.accessdata.fda.gov/scripts/cdrh/cfdocs/cfpma/pma.cfm?id=P210040.
57. Jänne PA, Riely GJ, Gadgeel SM, Heist RS, Ou SHI, Pacheco JM, et al. Adagrasib in non–small-cell lung cancer harboring a *KRAS*^{G12C} mutation. N Engl J Med. 2022;387(2):120–31.
58. Ou SHI, Jänne PA, Leal TA, Rybkin II, Sabari JK, Barve MA, et al. First-in-human phase I/IB dose-finding study of Adagrasib (MRTX849) in patients with advanced KRASG12C solid tumors (KRYSTAL-1). J Clin Oncol. 2022;40(23):2530–8.
59. Stitz R, Buder A, Silye R, Baumgartner B, Pühringer F, Filipits M, et al. Validation of a next-generation sequencing assay for the detection of EGFR mutations in cell-free circulating tumor DNA. Exp Mol Pathol. 2021;123:104685.

60. Stetson D, Ahmed A, Xu X, Nuttall BRB, Lubinski TJ, Johnson JH, et al. Orthogonal comparison of four plasma NGS tests with tumor suggests technical factors are a major source of assay discordance. JCO Precis Oncol. 2019;3:1–9.
61. Mack PC, Banks KC, Espenschied CR, Burich RA, Zill OA, Lee CE, et al. Spectrum of driver mutations and clinical impact of circulating tumor DNA analysis in non-small cell lung cancer: analysis of over 8000 cases. Cancer. 2020;126(14):3219–28.
62. Verma S, Moore MW, Ringler R, Ghosal A, Horvath K, Naef T, et al. Analytical performance evaluation of a commercial next generation sequencing liquid biopsy platform using plasma ctDNA, reference standards, and synthetic serial dilution samples derived from normal plasma. BMC Cancer. 2020;20(1):945.
63. Alborelli I, Generali D, Jermann P, Cappelletti MR, Ferrero G, Scaggiante B, et al. Cell-free DNA analysis in healthy individuals by next-generation sequencing: a proof of concept and technical validation study. Cell Death Dis. 2019;10(7):534.
64. Pritchett MA, Camidge DR, Patel M, Khatri J, Boniol S, Friedman EK, et al. Prospective clinical validation of the InVisionFirst-lung circulating tumor DNA assay for molecular profiling of patients with advanced nonsquamous non–small-cell lung cancer. JCO Precis Oncol. 2019;3:PO.18.00299.
65. Li BT, Janku F, Jung B, Hou C, Madwani K, Alden R, et al. Ultra-deep next-generation sequencing of plasma cell-free DNA in patients with advanced lung cancers: results from the Actionable Genome Consortium. Ann Oncol Off J Eur Soc Med Oncol [Internet]. 2019 [cited 2025 May 15];30(4). Available from: https://pubmed.ncbi.nlm.nih.gov/30891595/
66. Al Zoughbi W, Fox J, Beg S, Papp E, Hissong E, Ohara K, et al. Validation of a circulating tumor DNA-based next-generation sequencing assay in a cohort of patients with solid tumors: a proposed solution for decentralized plasma testing. Oncologist. 2021;26(11):e1971–81.
67. Truelsen D, Freire-Aradas A, Nazari M, Aliferi A, Ballard D, Phillips C, et al. Evaluation of a custom QIAseq targeted DNA panel with 164 ancestry informative markers sequenced with the Illumina MiSeq. Sci Rep. 2021;11(1):21040.
68. Li G, Pavlick D, Chung JH, Bauer T, Tan BA, Peguero J, et al. Genomic profiling of cell-free circulating tumor DNA in patients with colorectal cancer and its fidelity to the genomics of the tumor biopsy. J Gastrointest Oncol. 2019;10(5):831–40.
69. Zill OA, Banks KC, Fairclough SR, Mortimer SA, Vowles JV, Mokhtari R, et al. The landscape of actionable genomic alterations in cell-free circulating tumor DNA from 21,807 advanced cancer patients. Clin Cancer Res. 2018;24(15):3528–38.
70. Tukachinsky H, Madison RW, Chung JH, Gjoerup OV, Severson EA, Dennis L, et al. Genomic analysis of circulating tumor DNA in 3,334 patients with advanced prostate cancer identifies targetable BRCA alterations and AR resistance mechanisms. Clin Cancer Res. 2021;27(11):3094–105.
71. Kotecha RR, Gedvilaite E, Ptashkin R, Knezevic A, Murray S, Johnson I, et al. Matched molecular profiling of cell-free DNA and tumor tissue in patients with advanced clear cell renal cell carcinoma. JCO Precis Oncol. 2022;6:e2200012.
72. O'Leary B, Cutts RJ, Liu Y, Hrebien S, Huang X, Fenwick K, et al. The genetic landscape and clonal evolution of breast cancer resistance to Palbociclib plus Fulvestrant in the PALOMA-3 trial. Cancer Discov. 2018;8(11):1390–403.
73. Misale S, Yaeger R, Hobor S, Scala E, Janakiraman M, Liska D, et al. Emergence of KRAS mutations and acquired resistance to anti-EGFR therapy in colorectal cancer. Nature. 2012;486(7404):532–6.
74. Diaz LA Jr, Williams RT, Wu J, Kinde I, Hecht JR, Berlin J, et al. The molecular evolution of acquired resistance to targeted EGFR blockade in colorectal cancers. Nature. 2012;486(7404):537–40.
75. Bourrier C, Pierga JY, Xuereb L, Salaun H, Proudhon C, Speicher MR, et al. Shallow whole-genome sequencing from plasma identifies FGFR1 amplified breast cancers and predicts overall survival. Cancer. 2020;12(6):1481.
76. Antonarakis ES, Lu C, Wang H, Luber B, Nakazawa M, Roeser JC, et al. AR-V7 and resistance to enzalutamide and Abiraterone in prostate cancer. N Engl J Med. 2014;371(11):1028–38.
77. Scher HI, Graf RP, Schreiber NA, Jayaram A, Winquist E, McLaughlin B, et al. Assessment of the validity of nuclear-localized androgen receptor splice variant 7 in circulating tumor cells as a predictive biomarker for castration-resistant prostate cancer. JAMA Oncol. 2018;4(9):1179–86.
78. Armstrong AJ, Halabi S, Luo J, Nanus DM, Giannakakou P, Szmulewitz RZ, et al. Prospective multicenter validation of androgen receptor splice variant 7 and hormone therapy resistance in high-risk castration-resistant prostate cancer: the PROPHECY study. J Clin Oncol Off J Am Soc Clin Oncol. 2019;37(13):1120–9.
79. Ebright RY, Lee S, Wittner BS, Niederhoffer KL, Nicholson BT, Bardia A, et al. Deregulation of ribosomal protein expression and translation promotes breast cancer metastasis. Science. 2020;367(6485):1468–73.
80. Smerage JB, Barlow WE, Hortobagyi GN, Winer EP, Leyland-Jones B, Srkalovic G, et al. Circulating tumor cells and response to chemotherapy in metastatic breast cancer: SWOG S0500. J Clin Oncol Off J Am Soc Clin Oncol. 2014;32(31):3483–9.

Suggested Reading

Ultra-sensitive ctDNA mutation tracking to identify molecular residual disease and predict relapse in patients with early breast cancer. | J Clin Oncol [Internet]. [cited 2025 Apr 28]. Available from: https://ascopubs.org/doi/10.1200/JCO.2024.42.16_suppl.1010

6 Interpretation and Pitfalls in Liquid Biopsy

Liquid biopsy is a noninvasive diagnostic technology based on body fluids, including blood, and it is emerging as a promising approach that can overcome the limitations of conventional tissue biopsy by dynamically reflecting tumor-derived molecular information. In particular, liquid biopsy represents a significant turning point in the realization of precision oncology, as it can capture the spatial and temporal heterogeneity of cancer—that is, intratumoral clonal diversity and molecular evolution in response to therapy [1].

However, despite these technological advances, liquid biopsy is inherently based on biological materials (human-derived specimens) collected from an ex vivo, indirect environment, and thus, its interpretation is accompanied by unique limitations and complexities. Unlike tissue biopsy, which provides clear anatomical and pathological background information, liquid biopsy must extract meaningful signals from a mixture of diverse cellular and molecular components in the blood, a process in which the boundary between signal and noise can become ambiguous.

In practice, limitations in analytical sensitivity and specificity, biological heterogeneity and uneven distribution of analytes, lack of standardization across analytical platforms, and the potential for false-positive signals such as clonal hematopoiesis or background cfDNA have been consistently noted. These factors go beyond mere technical inconvenience and may lead to misinterpretation, unnecessary overtreatment, or delayed therapeutic opportunities, ultimately impacting the clinical utility of liquid biopsy. Therefore, this chapter systematically examines interpretive pitfalls that may be encountered in clinical and research settings, focusing on representative analytes such as ctDNA, CTCs, and EVs. The following sections sequentially address the following: ① the inherent limitations of the signal-to-noise ratio, ② strategies for interpreting low-concentration or undetectable signals, ③ the heterogeneity and standardization issues of EVs, ④ the clinical impact of cut-off and threshold settings, and ⑤ biological uncertainties based on indirect environments. By highlighting risk factors that are often overlooked in the interpretation of liquid biopsy results and comprehensively introducing scientific efforts and technical strategies to overcome these challenges, this chapter aims to provide readers with insights for more accurate and clinically meaningful interpretations.

6.1 Inherent Limitations of the Signal-to-Noise Ratio

Unlike traditional tissue biopsy, liquid biopsy is a noninvasive approach that captures the molecular characteristics of tumors based on analytes present in body fluids. However, one of the unavoidable inherent challenges is the limitation of the signal-to-noise ratio (SNR). This is a key factor

S. I. Kim, Y. Kim, *Liquid Biopsy for Cancer*, https://doi.org/10.1007/978-981-99-4418-7_6

that determines the diagnostic accuracy and clinical applicability of liquid biopsy results, and it is a prerequisite that must be considered during interpretation.

Most biomolecules in body fluids—cfDNA, EVs, proteins, circulating cells, etc.—are continuously produced and released even under normal physiological conditions, forming a certain background level. As a result, it can be difficult to distinguish whether a particular analyte represents a disease-associated pathological signal or merely physiological variation (noise). Since malignant tumors ultimately arise from transformed cell populations within host tissues, "tumor-specific signals that are entirely absent in the normal state" are extremely rare; most signals are interpreted based on their relative difference from normal signals. Therefore, isolating and quantifying low-abundance tumor-derived signals in a high-noise environment is a fundamental challenge faced by liquid biopsy technologies.

Clinically, in early-stage cancer or in postsurgical minimal residual disease, the tumor fraction is extremely low [2, 3]. No matter how much analytical sensitivity is increased, tumor-derived signals may be masked by noise, or conversely, non-tumor signals may be misinterpreted as tumor-derived, posing a significant risk. A representative example is CHIP (clonal hematopoiesis of indeterminate potential). CHIP is an age-related phenomenon involving the clonal expansion of hematopoietic cells with acquired mutations, commonly observed in genes such as TP53, DNMT3A, TET2, and ASXL1. These mutations can be present in plasma cfDNA and mistaken for tumor-derived mutations [4, 5, 6, 7]. Particularly in companion diagnostics, misinterpreting CHIP signals as cancer-related mutations can lead to unnecessary or inappropriate treatments, such as prescribing PARP inhibitors or immunotherapies. This is not merely a technical error but rather a clinical interpretive error with direct implications for patient safety, making it a serious concern.

To prevent this, recent recommendations include parallel analysis of paired WBC DNA to preemptively exclude CHIP-derived mutations. Additionally, some statistical correction methods utilize temporal patterns of VAF changes or gene-specific CHIP mutation frequencies. However, there is still no international consensus on cut-off values or interpretive criteria for CHIP discrimination, and results may vary depending on platform sensitivity and interpretive algorithms. Therefore, establishing an international diagnostic consensus based on large-scale prospective cohort data is essential in the future.

The issue of signal-to-noise ratio is not limited to cfDNA analysis. Interpretive pitfalls also exist in CTC analysis. For example, EpCAM-based positive selection strategies may result in false negatives if EpCAM expression is lost in cells that have undergone EMT (epithelial–mesenchymal transition). Conversely, if non-tumor inflammatory cells or cells derived from damaged tissue mimic CD45-negative, EpCAM-positive cells, this may lead to false-positive results. This is a representative example where the low abundance of CTCs in blood, their biological heterogeneity, and the limitations of isolation techniques collectively reduce the fidelity of the signal.

Similar issues have been reported with EVs. EVs are released not only from tumor cells but also from various normal cells such as platelets, erythrocytes, and leukocytes, resulting in an extremely heterogeneous plasma EV pool. In particular, distinguishing whether the protein or nucleic acid signals within EVs are "tumor-derived" or "normal-derived" requires highly sophisticated isolation and purification technologies, but currently, no standardized methods exist. Consequently, in EV research, non-tumor particles such as lipoproteins, protein aggregates, and platelet-derived vesicles are often co-isolated, leading to signal distortion. Therefore, in EV-based biomarker studies, the authenticity of the "signal" itself is always subject to debate, which starkly highlights the issue of SNR.

The inherent limitations of SNR thus go beyond mere technical constraints and are directly linked to the clinical interpretability and reliability of liquid biopsy results. Highly sensitive detection technologies may actually increase false positives and false negatives, leading to misdiagnosis, overtreatment, or treatment delays. Therefore, a thorough understanding of noise, sophisticated discrimination strategies, and rigorous clinical validation must be implemented in parallel. To control SNR and enhance interpretive reliability, it is essential to establish quantitative and qualitative quality control (QC) systems and to develop internationally standardized interpretive frameworks. Such efforts will be fundamental in elevating liquid biopsy from a research tool to a clinical standard.

6.2 Strategies for Interpreting Non-Detection or Low Abundance of Analytes

One of the most frequent challenges in the clinical interpretation of liquid biopsy is the situation where the analyte is "not detected" or present at "low abundance." In particular, ctDNA and CTCs may be present at extremely low concentrations or below the limit of detection in the blood, depending on pathological conditions or analytical parameters, making interpretations that rely solely on analytical sensitivity prone to clinical error.

ctDNA consists of DNA fragments released from tumor cells through apoptosis or necrosis, typically accounting for only a minute fraction (less than 0.01%) of total cfDNA [8, 9, 10]. Clinically, in early-stage cancers, postsurgical minimal residual disease, or tumors located in anatomical sites with limited blood flow such as the brain or bone, the release of ctDNA into the bloodstream is inherently low, a phenomenon referred to as non-shedding. Additionally, some tumors have low metabolic activity and limited vascularization, biologically restricting the production and release of ctDNA. In such cases, even with improved analytical sensitivity, detection may remain difficult or impossible.

Current technical approaches to address the low abundance of ctDNA include ultrasensitive NGS-based methods such as MAESTRO (mutation enrichment with specific hybridization and removal of off-targets) and TARDIS (targeted digital sequencing), as well as strategies involving serial sampling or simultaneous multi-target monitoring [11]. However, these technologies face limitations in terms of cost and turnaround time, restricting their widespread adoption in clinical practice.

Most importantly, non-detection of ctDNA does not necessarily indicate the absence of mutations. For example, in patients with non-small cell lung cancer (NSCLC) harboring EGFR mutations, a "not detected" result in ctDNA testing does not preclude the presence of the mutation, which may still be confirmed by tissue biopsy and serve as a basis for effective targeted therapy. Therefore, cfDNA results must always be interpreted in conjunction with the patient's clinical context, imaging findings, and pathology, and should be considered complementary rather than a replacement for tissue biopsy [12].

Circulating tumor cells (CTCs) are tumor cells present in the bloodstream and offer the advantage of providing information at the cellular level, but they are structurally limited in terms of analytical sensitivity. CTCs are rare, typically fewer than several dozen cells per milliliter of blood, making it challenging to isolate and enumerate a meaningful number from just a few milliliters of blood, which is a technically very challenging task. Moreover, there is still a lack of universal interpretive criteria that can define the causal relationship between the presence of CTCs and clinical events (e.g., recurrence, treatment resistance). The cut-off values based on CTC counts also vary depending on the cancer type, and in many cases, there are no quantified guidelines for interpreting pre- and posttreatment changes [13, 14]. As a result, interpretation of CTC-based liquid biopsy must be approached multidimensionally in conjunction with the clinical context, and longitudinal analysis for individual patients should be performed in parallel to ensure clinical relevance.

In EV analysis as well, issues of low concentration or non-detection are significant. Since EVs are released from normal cells such as platelets, erythrocytes, and leukocytes, the proportion of tumor-derived EVs within total plasma EVs is extremely low. Therefore, if tumor-specific EVs cannot be isolated, the signal is often masked by noise or may not be detected at all. Recently, immunoaffinity-based isolation methods, microfluidic chips, and nanowire platforms have been investigated to enrich tumor-derived EVs, but clinical standardization has not yet been achieved.

Given these practical limitations, the clinical application of liquid biopsy is most appropriate in situations where tissue biopsy is not feasible, repeated biopsies are limited due to patient condition, or in areas where longitudinal monitoring such as treatment response and recurrence tracking is critical. For liquid biopsy to be used as an independent diagnostic tool at initial diagnosis, it must provide sufficient biological reliability and analytical sensitivity to predict the presence of disease beyond mere detection of analytes. At present, this is only feasible for certain cancer types and high-risk patient groups.

6.3 Heterogeneity of EVs and Lack of Standardization

Extracellular vesicles (EVs) are nanoscale vesicles secreted by living cells that circulate in body fluids, contributing to intercellular signaling and the transport of biomolecules. They are detected in various body fluids such as blood, urine, saliva, and cerebrospinal fluid, and they contain proteins, nucleic acids, and lipids that reflect the molecular characteristics of their parent cells. Thus, they are considered potential biomarkers that mirror the pathological or physiological state of cells. Owing to these properties, EVs have attracted attention as key analytes in liquid biopsy.

However, EVs are not a single entity but a heterogeneous population composed of different subtypes according to size, biogenesis pathway, and cell of origin [15, 16]. Typically, they are classified as (1) small EVs (sEVs, <200 nm), which are endosome-derived vesicles released via fusion of multivesicular bodies (MVBs) with the plasma membrane, and (2) large EVs (lEVs, >200 nm), which include microvesicles and apoptotic bodies generated by outward budding of the plasma membrane or during cell death. However, these distinctions are merely convenient classifications based on size; in actual physiological conditions, size ranges overlap and biogenesis pathways are mixed, making it difficult to use these as definitive criteria. Furthermore, a single cell can simultaneously release multiple EV subtypes, and their composition changes dynamically depending on cell state, stimuli, and the tumor microenvironment (TME). In particular, in solid tumors, intratumoral heterogeneity is reflected at the EV level, resulting in a highly diverse mixture of EVs according to malignancy, metabolic state, and treatment responsiveness.

In addition to this biological heterogeneity, technical heterogeneity is also a significant issue. The most widely used EV isolation method to date is ultracentrifugation (UC), which is limited by low yield, long processing times, and the requirement for large sample volumes. Moreover, it cannot completely eliminate contamination by non-EV co-isolates such as cell debris, protein complexes, and lipoproteins. Recently, new technologies such as size-exclusion chromatography (SEC), immunoaffinity capture, and microfluidic-based platforms have emerged, but each method tends to be selectively biased toward specific EV subtypes. Consequently, even with samples from the same patient, different isolation methods may yield divergent results. This complicates the comparison between studies. Decreased feasibility and reproducibility severely hinder clinical translatability.

A more clinically significant issue is the lack of evidence regarding which EV subtypes truly represent tumor characteristics. While small EVs are known to reliably reflect the molecular information of parent cells, there are also reports that large EVs can accurately indicate tumor origin under certain conditions. Some studies have detected driver mutations, copy number alterations, and tumor-specific proteins in oncosomes or large EVs. Thus, the correlation between EV size-based classification and tumor specificity remains unclear.

To address this confusion, the International Society for Extracellular Vesicles (ISEV) released the revised MISEV (Minimal Information for Studies of Extracellular Vesicles) guidelines in 2023 [17]. MISEV2023 recommends avoiding the indiscriminate use of the term "exosome" in

EV nomenclature and discourages its application to vesicles of unknown origin. The guidelines also mandate transparent reporting of EV isolation and purification methods, specification of a minimal biomarker panel for EV characterization (such as TSG101, ALIX, CD9, CD63, and CD81), experimental design under equivalent conditions, and reporting of negative controls as essential criteria. Nevertheless, researchers continue to independently apply various techniques, and the lack of standardized isolation and purification protocols remains one of the major obstacles to reproducibility and clinical translation in EV research. In particular, for regulatory approval, protocol standardization, quantitative interpretation criteria, and a quality control (QC) system are essential.

Current active efforts include (1) identification of molecular markers distinguishing EV biogenesis pathways, (2) discovery of cell type-specific EV markers, (3) functional analysis of EV cargo (e.g., miRNA, lncRNA, DNA, proteins), and (4) development of high-purity isolation technologies. Some studies subdivide EVs into exosome-like vesicles, ectosomes, and oncosomes to explore functional differences, while high-resolution flow cytometry, single-particle interferometric imaging, electrokinetic isolation, and label-free spectroscopic analysis are being proposed as novel quantitative and qualitative tools. Furthermore, multi-omics approaches combining proteomics, transcriptomics, and lipidomics are playing an increasingly important role in elucidating the functional characteristics of EV subtypes.

In conclusion, EV-based liquid biopsy still faces the fundamental question: "Which EVs are truly tumor-derived?" This is not merely a basic research issue, but a core challenge directly linked to clinical translation, regulatory approval, and ultimately the realization of precision medicine. Moving forward, comparative studies among EV subtypes, determination of their origins, standardization of high-purity isolation techniques, establishment of analytical algorithms, and integrated standardization efforts led by international consortia must proceed in parallel. With such efforts, EVs could stand alongside ctDNA and CTCs as an independent pillar of precision liquid biopsy.

6.4 Clinical Impact of Cut-Off and Threshold Determination

One of the most distinctive features of liquid biopsy is its ability to provide quantitative results. The frequency of specific genetic mutations, the number of circulating tumor cells in the blood, or the expression levels of particular proteins and nucleic acids contained in extracellular vesicles can all be expressed numerically, and these values are directly linked to clinical decision-making. However, every quantitative result inevitably requires the establishment of a threshold, or cut-off value. The challenge is that this value is not merely a numerical boundary, but serves as a critical reference point that determines patient treatment strategies and prognosis.

For example, in the case of circulating tumor cells (CTCs), the CellSearch system defines the presence of five or more CTCs in 7.5 mL of blood as being associated with poor prognosis [18]. But in actual clinical practice, can a patient with four CTCs simply be interpreted as negative? The clinical significance of a single-cell difference in terms of patient survival and treatment strategy goes beyond a simple statistical distinction. This case clearly demonstrates that the cut-off is not merely an experimental criterion, but a critical variable in the interpretation of patient diagnosis and treatment.

Threshold values should be set differently depending on the purpose of the test. In cases where the goal is early diagnosis or large-scale cancer screening, it is important to minimize overdiagnosis, unnecessary testing, and the resulting economic and psychological burdens caused by false positives. Therefore, in such situations, a higher threshold prioritizing specificity is often chosen, which inevitably leads to some patients being classified as false negatives. In fact, multi-cancer early detection platforms report a positive result only when a specific DNA methylation signal exceeds a certain threshold, and their strategies are designed to maximize positive predictive value [19].

Conversely, in situations such as postsurgical residual disease surveillance or monitoring of treatment response, it is essential to detect even the lowest possible signal, making sensitivity the top priority. In these cases, a very low threshold is applied. State-of-the-art ctDNA-based platforms such as RaDaR™ and Signatera™ are designed to detect extremely low variant allele frequencies, below 0.01%, enabling the detection of recurrence before radiological evidence appears.

However, the same numerical value does not always carry the same meaning. For example, a 0.2% KRAS mutation may serve as a critical basis for therapeutic intervention in early-stage colorectal cancer patients, but in patients with advanced cancer and high tumor burden, it may be regarded as a mere background signal. Similarly, the presence of fewer than five CTCs cannot be taken as definitive evidence of a favorable prognosis. Without a comprehensive consideration of cancer type, stage, treatment history, and accompanying clinical findings, simple numerical interpretation can lead to false negatives or interpretive errors. Ultimately, the cut-off is not a fixed absolute value, but a relative criterion that must be reinterpreted within the clinical context.

The problem is that, to this day, cut-off criteria still vary widely depending on the analytical platform, cancer type, and indication. In cfDNA analysis, detection sensitivity differs among ddPCR, BEAMing, and NGS panels, and even samples from the same patient can yield different results depending on the platform. CTC analysis also applies different thresholds depending on the technique, such as CellSearch, microfluidic systems, or size-based separation methods. These inconsistencies hinder the comparison of research results, complicate the interpretation of multicenter clinical trial data, and pose a major obstacle to clinical standardization.

To address these issues, several improvements are needed. First, a cross-validation system should be established to compare and calibrate results across different platforms. In addition, detailed guidelines are required to set context-specific criteria according to cancer type, stage, and treatment phase. Furthermore, it is important to develop dynamic threshold models that reflect individual patient characteristics and temporal changes, based on large-scale patient data accumulated in real-world clinical settings. Integrating data from multiple analytes (ctDNA, CTC, EV, etc.) using artificial intelligence and machine learning, and generating risk scores instead of relying on simple absolute values, represents a promising approach in this direction. In radiology, AI-based interpretation systems have already demonstrated improved diagnostic accuracy by optimizing the balance between sensitivity and specificity, and this approach is fully applicable to liquid biopsy interpretation as well [20, 21].

Ultimately, the threshold is not a technical choice but an extension of clinical judgment. Its determination and interpretation are directly linked to patient prognosis and therefore must be based not on simple numerical values, but on a comprehensive understanding of the patient's condition and context, the characteristics of the analytical technology, and accumulated clinical data. With the future introduction of international standardization and AI-based precision interpretation tools, the threshold will evolve from a rigid number into a real-time indicator enabling truly personalized precision medicine.

6.5 Fundamental Limitations: Biological Uncertainty

Unlike tissue biopsy, which involves direct sampling of the tumor or microscopic visualization, liquid biopsy infers the presence and characteristics of a tumor indirectly by analyzing molecular traces dispersed in the bloodstream or bodily fluids. This feature enables the key advantages of liquid biopsy—its noninvasiveness and the possibility of repeated measurements—but it also inherently introduces uncertainty in the interpretation process. In other words, rather than observing tumor cells themselves, we are interpreting the molecular "echoes" left behind by these cells. Unless there is robust biological evidence that these echoes faithfully reflect tumor biology, no quantitative analysis based solely on such signals should be considered clinically definitive.

In particular, circulating analytes such as ctDNA, CTCs, and EVs can also be released by normal cells under various physiological and pathological conditions. Therefore, if it cannot be scientifically demonstrated that a given signal truly originates from a tumor, the results may be meaningless or lead to serious misinterpretation. A representative example is clonal hematopoiesis of indeterminate potential (CHIP), a phenomenon in which blood cells acquire mutations in genes such as TP53, DNMT3A, and TET2 with aging. These mutations can be misinterpreted as tumor-derived mutations in ctDNA analysis. In fact, there is concern that CHIP-derived mutations have been mistaken for cancer-related mutations in some patients, leading to unnecessary administration of PARP inhibitors or immunotherapies. The same issue arises in CTC detection: if nonmalignant epithelial cells are captured or if nonspecific binding occurs in EpCAM-based assays, they may be misclassified as CTCs, resulting in false-positive interpretations for patients. The situation is similar in EV research. Since plasma EVs originate from a variety of cells, including platelets, leukocytes, and erythrocytes, failure to enrich tumor-specific EVs can yield analyses that primarily reflect background noise rather than tumor biology.

Given these characteristics, liquid biopsy should not generally be used in isolation to provide a definitive interpretation. Clinical information such as disease stage, anatomical location of the tumor, imaging findings, histological subtype, and treatment history must be integrated. For example, in patients with bone metastases as the main lesion, the absence of detectable ctDNA may simply reflect a low amount of DNA released into the bloodstream, rather than the absence of recurrence. Therefore, complementary interpretation with imaging findings or tissue-based analyses is necessary. Similarly, in EV analysis, if it cannot be determined that a particular vesicle is truly tumor-derived, even high quantitative values cannot be assigned clinical significance. Ultimately, liquid biopsy is fundamentally limited by its indirect assessment of the tumor environment.

In this context, the interpretation of liquid biopsy always requires a high level of critical thinking and understanding of the clinical context. The limitations discussed in this chapter—such as the signal-to-noise ratio, low analyte concentrations, heterogeneity and lack of standardization in EVs, and uncertainty in threshold settings—are representative pitfalls encountered in the interpretation of liquid biopsy. These are not merely technical obstacles, but stem from the fact that liquid biopsy inherently deals with indirect and incomplete biological information. Therefore, the future of liquid biopsy will not be achieved simply by increasing the sensitivity and specificity of detection technologies.

To achieve true clinical value, first, basic research is needed to clarify the origin of analytes and their association with disease; second, interpretation algorithms and analytical criteria must be refined to reduce false positives and false negatives; and third, integrated interpretive guidelines that reflect the clinical context must be established. When scientific rigor, biological reliability, and clinical appropriateness converge, liquid biopsy can become a core tool of patient-centered precision medicine, rather than merely an auxiliary diagnostic method. Ultimately, it is this very uncertainty and the ongoing efforts to overcome it that elevate liquid biopsy from a simple methodology to a transformative shift in the medical paradigm. It eloquently attests to a leading journey.

References

1. Heitzer E, Haque IS, Roberts CES, Speicher MR. Current and future perspectives of liquid biopsies in genomics-driven oncology. Nat Rev Genet. 2019;20(2):71–88.
2. Gale D, Heider K, Ruiz-Valdepenas A, Hackinger S, Perry M, Marsico G, et al. Residual ctDNA after treatment predicts early relapse in patients with early-stage non-small cell lung cancer. Ann Oncol. 2022;33(5):500–10.
3. Semenkovich NP, Szymanski JJ, Earland N, Chauhan PS, Pellini B, Chaudhuri AA. Genomic approaches

to cancer and minimal residual disease detection using circulating tumor DNA. J Immunother Cancer. 2023;11(6):e006284.
4. Chan HT, Chin YM, Nakamura Y, Low SK. Clonal hematopoiesis in liquid biopsy: from biological noise to valuable clinical implications. Cancer. 2020;12(8):2277.
5. Bernard E, Micol JB. CHIP'ing signal from noise in liquid biopsy. Clin Cancer Res. 2025;31(13):2545–6.
6. Genovese G, Kähler AK, Handsaker RE, Lindberg J, Rose SA, Bakhoum SF, et al. Clonal hematopoiesis and blood-cancer risk inferred from blood DNA sequence. N Engl J Med. 2014;371(26):2477–87.
7. Jaiswal S, Fontanillas P, Flannick J, Manning A, Grauman PV, Mar BG, et al. Age-related clonal hematopoiesis associated with adverse outcomes. N Engl J Med. 2014;371(26):2488–98.
8. Sánchez-Herrero E, Serna-Blasco R, Robado de Lope L, González-Rumayor V, Romero A, Provencio M. Circulating tumor DNA as a cancer biomarker: an overview of biological features and factors that may impact on ctDNA analysis. Front Oncol. 2022;12:943253.
9. Panet F, Papakonstantinou A, Borrell M, Vivancos J, Vivancos A, Oliveira M. Use of ctDNA in early breast cancer: analytical validity and clinical potential. NPJ Breast Cancer. 2024;10(1):50.
10. Sassorossi C, Evangelista J, Stefani A, Chiappetta M, Martino A, Campanella A, et al. The role of ctDNA for diagnosis and histological prediction in early stage non-small-cell lung cancer: a narrative review. Diagnostics. 2025;15(7):904.
11. Sim ES, Rhoades J, Xiong K, Walsh L, Crnjac A, Blewett T, et al. Immediate postoperative minimal residual disease detection with MAESTRO predicts recurrence and survival in head and neck cancer patients treated with surgery [Internet]. medRxiv. 2025 [cited 2025 Sep 8]:2025.01.27.25321202. Available from: https://www.medrxiv.org/content/10.1101/2025.01.27.25321202v1.
12. Merker JD, Oxnard GR, Compton C, Diehn M, Hurley P, Lazar AJ, et al. Circulating tumor DNA analysis in patients with cancer: American Society of Clinical Oncology and College of American Pathologists Joint Review. J Clin Oncol [Internet]. 2018 [cited 2025 Apr 29]. Available from: https://ascopubs.org/doi/10.1200/JCO.2017.76.8671.
13. de Bono JS, Scher HI, Montgomery RB, Parker C, Miller MC, Tissing H, et al. Circulating tumor cells predict survival benefit from treatment in metastatic castration-resistant prostate cancer. Clin Cancer Res. 2008;14(19):6302–9.
14. Cohen SJ, Punt CJA, Iannotti N, Saidman BH, Sabbath KD, Gabrail NY, et al. Relationship of circulating tumor cells to tumor response, progression-free survival, and overall survival in patients with metastatic colorectal cancer. J Clin Oncol. 2008;26(19):3213–21.
15. van de Wakker SI, Meijers FM, Sluijter JPG, Vader P. Extracellular vesicle heterogeneity and its impact for regenerative medicine applications. Pharmacol Rev. 2023;75(5):1043–61.
16. Willms E, Cabañas C, Mäger I, Wood MJA, Vader P. Extracellular vesicle heterogeneity: subpopulations, isolation techniques, and diverse functions in cancer progression. Front Immunol [Internet]. 2018 [cited 2025 Sep 8];9. Available from: https://www.frontiersin.org/journals/immunology/articles/10.3389/fimmu.2018.00738/full.
17. Zhang Y, Lan M, Chen Y. Minimal information for studies of extracellular vesicles (MISEV): ten-year evolution (2014–2023). Pharmaceutics. 2024;16(11):1394.
18. Cristofanilli M, Budd GT, Ellis MJ, Stopeck A, Matera J, Miller MC, et al. Circulating tumor cells, disease progression, and survival in metastatic breast cancer. N Engl J Med. 2004;351(8):781–91.
19. Liu MC, Oxnard GR, Klein EA, Swanton C, Seiden MV, Liu MC, et al. Sensitive and specific multi-cancer detection and localization using methylation signatures in cell-free DNA. Ann Oncol. 2020;31(6):745–59.
20. McKinney SM, Sieniek M, Godbole V, Godwin J, Antropova N, Ashrafian H, et al. International evaluation of an AI system for breast cancer screening. Nature. 2020;577(7788):89–94.
21. Ardila D, Kiraly AP, Bharadwaj S, Choi B, Reicher JJ, Peng L, et al. End-to-end lung cancer screening with three-dimensional deep learning on low-dose chest computed tomography. Nat Med. 2019;25(6):954–61.

Suggested Reading

Yu DD, Wu Y, Shen HY, Lv MM, Chen WX, Zhang XH, et al. Exosomes in development, metastasis and drug resistance of breast cancer. Cancer Sci. 2015;106(8):959–64.

Castro-Giner F, Gkountela S, Donato C, Alborelli I, Quagliata L, Ng CKY, et al. Cancer diagnosis using a liquid biopsy: challenges and expectations. Diagn Basel Switz. 2018;8(2):31.

Moser T, Kühberger S, Lazzeri I, Vlachos G, Heitzer E. Bridging biological cfDNA features and machine learning approaches. Trends Genet TIG. 2023;39(4):285–307.

Bu A, Wu G, Hu L. Revealing the heterogeneity of extracellular vesicles: from population to single particle level. Proteomics [Internet]. [cited 2025 Sep 8]. Available from: https://onlinelibrary.wiley.com/doi/abs/10.1002/pmic.70024.

De Sousa KP, Rossi I, Abdullahi M, Ramirez MI, Stratton D, Inal JM. Isolation and characterization of extracellular vesicles and future directions in diagnosis and therapy. Wiley Interdiscip Rev Nanomed Nanobiotechnol. 2023;15(1):e1835.

Bellotti C, Lang K, Kuplennik N, Sosnik A, Steinfeld R. High-grade extracellular vesicles preparation by combined size-exclusion and affinity chromatography. Sci Rep. 2021;11(1):10550.

Welsh JA, van der Pol E, Bettin BA, Carter DRF, Hendrix A, Lenassi M, et al. Towards defining reference materials for measuring extracellular vesicle refractive index, epitope abundance, size and concentration. J Extracell Vesicles. 2020;9(1):1816641.

Reinert T, Henriksen TV, Christensen E, Sharma S, Salari R, Sethi H, et al. Analysis of plasma cell-free DNA by ultradeep sequencing in patients with stages I to III colorectal cancer. JAMA Oncol. 2019;5(8):1124–31.

Chaudhuri AA, Chabon JJ, Lovejoy AF, Newman AM, Stehr H, Azad TD, et al. Early detection of molecular residual disease in localized lung cancer by circulating tumor DNA profiling. Cancer Discov. 2017;7(12):1394–403.

Newman AM, Lovejoy AF, Klass DM, Kurtz DM, Chabon JJ, Scherer F, et al. Integrated digital error suppression for improved detection of circulating tumor DNA. Nat Biotechnol. 2016;34(5):547–55.

Circulating Immune Biomarkers 7

Tumors evade immune surveillance through various mechanisms, including genetic mutations, dynamic changes in the tumor microenvironment, and activation of immune suppression and escape pathways. The primary goal of tumor immunotherapy is to inhibit these immune evasion mechanisms, thereby exposing tumor cells to the patient's immune system and activating immune responses against the tumor, ultimately inducing tumor cell death. The ultimate aim is to selectively eliminate tumor cells without affecting normal cells. These mechanisms have been clinically validated since the 2010s and are now established as standard treatment options for many solid tumors.

Immune checkpoint inhibitors (ICIs) function by inhibiting proteins that are involved in downregulating immune responses, thereby blocking immune escape mechanisms. This allows the immune system to recognize tumors, which have disguised themselves as self, as nonself, and exposes them to the patient's immune environment, leading to tumor cell death. Since the first approval of ipilimumab, targeting CTLA-4, in 2011, a series of agents have been approved, including nivolumab, pembrolizumab, and cemiplimab targeting PD-1, as well as atezolizumab, avelumab, and durvalumab targeting PD-L1. These immunotherapeutic agents have been applied across a wide range of malignancies. Notably, by 2020, seven ICIs had received FDA and EMA approval. In 2024, the PD-1 inhibitor tislelizumab was formally approved for gastric and gastroesophageal junction adenocarcinoma, marking the ninth immune checkpoint inhibitor to enter clinical practice. Recent reports indicate that the global ICI market continues to grow at a double-digit annual rate, and ICIs are expanding their indications beyond solid tumors to include hematologic malignancies and rare cancers.

In particular, the Keynote-024 and -189 clinical trials demonstrated significant improvements in overall survival (OS) in patients with advanced and metastatic non-small cell lung cancer (NSCLC) treated with pembrolizumab, either as monotherapy or in combination with chemotherapy [1]. The 5-year follow-up of Keynote-024 reported a median OS of 26.3 months, nearly double that of the chemotherapy group (13.4 months) [2]. Additionally, Keynote-189 showed that the combination group reduced the risk of death by approximately 51% compared to chemotherapy alone, establishing immune checkpoint inhibitors not merely as effective for select patient populations but as a paradigm-shifting strategy in clinical oncology [3]. These achievements have ushered in a new era of cancer treatment, known as the immuno-oncology era.

However, a detailed analysis of clinical trial results reveals that, even within the same cancer type and with the same therapeutic agent, there is a clear distinction between responders and nonresponders. For example, in Keynote-024, some patients with high PD-L1 expression did not respond, while long-term survivors were observed even among those with low expression.

S. I. Kim, Y. Kim, *Liquid Biopsy for Cancer*, https://doi.org/10.1007/978-981-99-4418-7_7

This heterogeneity underscores the necessity for predictive biomarkers in ICI therapy. In fact, various biomarkers such as PD-L1, TMB, and MSI-H/dMMR have been proposed and applied during the approval process for immune checkpoint inhibitors, but no single marker has yet been able to fully predict therapeutic response. Therefore, this chapter will review the limitations of existing tissue-based biomarkers and comprehensively examine the potential and latest research findings on liquid biopsy-based circulating immune biomarkers (Fig. 7.1).

To implement immunotherapy, it is essential to select appropriate treatments based on the molecular biological characteristics of the tumor and the features of the tumor immune microenvironment, as well as to accurately predict prognosis. The use and evaluation of biomarkers are necessary. Currently, the only predictive biomarker for ICI is the measurement of PD-L1 expression in tumor tissue sections using immunohistochemistry (IHC) staining. In most cases, this is used as a pathological assessment criterion, but PD-L1 as a biomarker has technical and biological limitations. Specifically, since PD-L1 is expressed in both immune cells and tumor cells, evaluating therapeutic efficacy can become complex. Furthermore, the degree of PD-L1 expression varies within the tumor itself, so a biopsy that samples only a small portion of the tumor may not be representative of the entire tumor [4]. As a result, patients whose biopsy is taken from a region with low expression may be excluded from treatment, even if they are eligible, leading to missed opportunities for appropriate therapy. Recent meta-analyses have also reported that PD-L1 IHC shows considerable variability in sensitivity and specificity and that correlation coefficients differ depending on the test kit and interpretation criteria. This highlights why PD-L1 is currently regarded in clinical practice as an "imperfect but usable biomarker." In addition to PD-L1, tumor mutational burden (TMB) detected in tumor tissue has recently

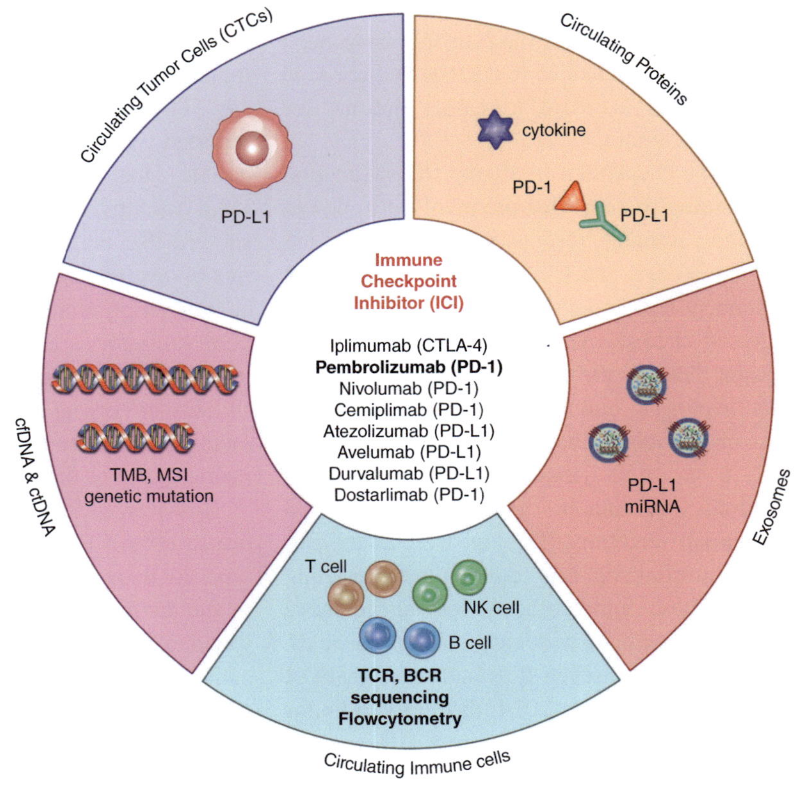

Fig. 7.1 Circulating immune markers for immune checkpoint inhibitor therapy

emerged as a novel biomarker for immunotherapy across various cancers. TMB reflects the genetic characteristics of the tumor, as tumor cells accumulate more genetic mutations than normal cells. These mutations can increase the aggressiveness of tumor cells and induce resistance to targeted therapies. However, cells with a high number of such mutations are more likely to be recognized as nonself, potentially resulting in a higher response rate to immunotherapy. TMB can be measured by sequencing tumor tissue obtained from a biopsy using next-generation sequencing (NGS) and is evaluated as the number of mutations per megabase (mutation/Mb) within a defined region of DNA. The value of TMB was confirmed in a prospective study evaluating the efficacy of nivolumab plus ipilimumab combination therapy in NSCLC patients, which demonstrated improved immunotherapy outcomes in advanced NSCLC, and similar results have been observed in other solid tumors. However, before TMB can be applied in clinical practice, experimental standardization as well as clinical and technical validation are required. Based on the Keynote-158 study, the FDA approved pembrolizumab in 2020 for the treatment of patients with unresectable or metastatic solid tumors with TMB-high (≥10 mut/Mb), demonstrating its potential utility as a biomarker for immunotherapy. Recently, blood-based TMB (bTMB) analysis has also been attempted, and evidence from studies such as the POPLAR (NCT01903993) and OAK (NCT02912559) derived cohorts, as well as the B-F1RST study (NCT02848651), suggests that bTMB can predict response independently of PD-L1 expression, positioning it as a leading candidate for future liquid biopsy-based immune biomarkers. Furthermore, in 2017, the FDA approved pembrolizumab for the treatment of patients with solid tumors exhibiting high microsatellite instability (MSI-H) or mismatch repair deficiency (dMMR), marking the first instance of a biomarker-based approval regardless of cancer type. When there is a genetic defect in the mismatch repair (MMR) proteins, which are responsible for correcting errors during DNA replication, errors accumulate in the short repetitive sequences of DNA known as microsatellites, resulting in high instability (MSI-H). In a study involving 90 patients with metastatic colorectal cancer and 59 patients with 14 other cancer types, all confirmed to have these characteristics by PCR and IHC, pembrolizumab treatment resulted in an overall survival rate of 39.6% and a complete response rate of 7%. More recently, dostarlimab received approval in February 2023 for the treatment of recurrent or advanced endometrial cancer with dMMR. Furthermore, in 2024, dostarlimab attracted significant attention in the academic community by demonstrating a 100% complete response rate in patients with locally advanced rectal cancer, highlighting that immune checkpoint inhibitors can achieve unprecedented outcomes in specific biomarker-defined populations. This case suggests the potential of fundamentally reshaping current therapeutic strategies.

Despite the remarkable improvement in ICI treatment response rates achieved through the identification and application of such biomarkers, many challenges remain. The limitations of these assays are, first, that PD-L1 expression assessed by IHC, as well as MSI and TMB evaluations, are tissue-based analyses that rely on small biopsy samples, which may not be representative of the entire tumor. Additionally, the low proportion of tumor cells in the biopsy may render analysis impossible. Second, even among patients with high TMB, MSI, and PD-L1 expression in tumor cells, immunotherapy may fail in some cases, while, conversely, patients with low expression may exhibit high response rates to immunotherapy. In fact, recent multicenter retrospective analyses have reported ICI response rates of 10–20% even in the PD-L1 negative group, with some patients achieving long-term survival. This demonstrates that a single biomarker alone is insufficient to fully capture or predict treatment response. Therefore, to overcome these limitations, the development of more robust biomarkers is required, and new approaches to existing biomarkers are also necessary. Third, these biomarkers should be continuously assessable throughout the course of treatment, and sample acquisition should not pose significant challenges. Finally, as tumors may adapt to therapeutic strategies and develop resistance, repeated monitoring must be feasible to enable timely and appropriate therapeutic adjustments. Most current assays provide static (baseline) information based on pretreatment biopsies. However, immune responses are highly dynamic, and the tumor microenvironment continuously evolves during therapy. Thus, biomarkers should be repeatedly evaluated during and after treatment. Recent prospective cohort studies have shown that clearance of blood-based ctDNA at 6 weeks after treatment initiation, dynamic changes in exosomal PD-L1, and peripheral TCR diversity have been shown to be closely associated with treatment response, supporting the clinical value of serial liquid biopsies.

For these reasons, liquid biopsy is being considered the most appropriate method for measuring immunotherapy biomarkers, and active research is underway to develop predictive biomarkers using liquid biopsy across various cancers. As previously described, liquid biopsy is minimally invasive, is cost-effective, and provides rapid information to clinicians making therapeutic decisions. In particular, it enables the detection of minimal residual disease (MRD) and mechanisms of resistance to therapy, which are not possible with tissue biopsy, and can be easily repeated during treatment without burdening the patient. Furthermore, its rapid turnaround allows for timely adjustments in therapeutic strategy based on treatment response. Recently, large-scale prospective clinical trials have reported that liquid biopsy-based ctDNA dynamics can predict ICI response early and detect the emergence of resistance mutations before they are visible on imaging, thereby increasing the feasibility of clinical application.

As described above, liquid biopsy most commonly utilizes body fluids, especially blood, but depending on tumor type, pleural fluid, saliva, cerebrospinal fluid, and urine may also be used. Efforts are underway to use components such as circulating cell-free DNA (cfDNA), particularly circulating tumor DNA (ctDNA), and circulating tumor cells (CTCs), as well as proteins, extracellular vesicles, and especially exosomes, as biomarkers for immunotherapy. Recently, the clinical value of circulating protein biomarkers such as serum IL-8, IFN-γ, and soluble PD-L1 has been reported, expanding the scope of liquid biopsy-based immune biomarkers beyond simple tumor DNA detection to encompass the broader immune system.

Body fluids such as blood contain large numbers of immune cells, including T cells and B cells, which can also be analyzed through liquid biopsy. Recently, through the analysis of these immune cell characteristics, various studies are being conducted to utilize them as diagnostic, therapeutic, and prognostic biomarkers for the implementation of immunotherapy. The tumor microenvironment (TME) is composed of tumor cells, cancer-associated fibroblasts (CAFs), various immune cells, and the extracellular matrix (ECM). Depending on the dynamic interactions among these cells, diverse mechanisms such as tumor survival, proliferation, and metastasis occur. Immune checkpoint inhibitors influence the TME, ultimately leading to the inhibition of tumor growth and induction of tumor cell death. Recent studies have demonstrated that a significant proportion of gene clonality is shared between tumor-infiltrating lymphocytes (TILs) in the TME and peripheral blood immune cells, suggesting that TCR sequencing of peripheral blood may serve as a surrogate marker for tumor immune responses. Therefore, understanding the tumor microenvironment is crucial for effective immunotherapy. A recent study reported that T cell receptor (TCR) clones of T cells within the breast cancer TME are largely shared with those in peripheral blood, indicating that they may reflect the antigen specificity of tumor cells. Other studies have also revealed that immune cells from tumor samples and those in peripheral blood share clonality, suggesting that the specificity of immune cells present in the TME is mirrored by those in peripheral blood. Based on these findings, in addition to classical liquid biopsy methods such as CTCs, cfDNA, exosomes, and plasma proteins, approaches utilizing immune cells—particularly T cells—in peripheral blood are emerging. These methods are likely to become important tools for predicting ICI responsiveness and monitoring resistance in the future.

7.1 Candidate Immune Markers for Liquid Biopsy

7.1.1 Circulating Tumor Cells (CTCs)

Circulating tumor cells (CTCs) have potential utility for predicting and monitoring the therapeutic response to immune checkpoint inhibitors (ICIs). The expression of immune checkpoint proteins such as PD-1, PD-L1, and CTLA-4 changes dynamically according to interactions between the tumor microenvironment and immune cells, and tissue biopsy-based detection of immune biomarkers may not adequately reflect this heterogeneity and spatial limitation. Consequently, CTC-based liquid biopsy is being proposed as a complementary approach to assess the systemic immune characteristics of tumors. Large-scale prospective studies published in 2022 and 2023 have reported that PD-L1 expression in CTCs is significantly correlated with ICI responsiveness in NSCLC patients and that a subset of responders can be identified even among patients with PD-L1-negative tumors by tissue analysis.

PD-L1 expression on CTCs has been reported in various cancer types and is attracting attention as a biomarker for predicting response to immune checkpoint inhibitors. For example, in metastatic breast cancer, non-small cell lung cancer (NSCLC), and prostate cancer, PD-L1-positive CTCs sometimes show results that differ from tissue-based PD-L1 expression, suggesting that CTCs may more precisely reflect the spatial heterogeneity of tumors. In a recent small-scale clinical study, a decrease in circulating PD-L1+ CTCs was associated with improved progression-free survival (PFS) in patients treated with pembrolizumab, whereas persistent detection of PD-L1+ CTCs was interpreted as indicative of therapeutic resistance [5].

The EpCAM-based immunomagnetic separation method is a representative technology for isolating CTCs, effectively separating CTCs that express epithelial cell markers. However, in CTCs that have undergone epithelial-to-mesenchymal transition (EMT), EpCAM expression is reduced; thus, this method may fail to capture CTCs in the EMT state. EMT CTCs are highly invasive and metastatic and often exhibit increased PD-L1 expression. Thus, missing their detection can result in a significant loss of critical information. Recent studies have developed dual-marker-based chips capable of simultaneously detecting EMT markers, demonstrating that PD-L1 expression can be successfully analyzed even in EpCAM-negative CTCs. To overcome these limitations, antigen-independent separation technologies such as cell size-based filtration and microfluidic systems have been developed. CellSieve™ is one such technology, enabling the efficient isolation of multiple CTC subtypes and cancer-associated macrophage-like cells (CAMLs) [6]. For example, in a study involving 41 NSCLC patients, the CellSieve™ filter was used to isolate EMT CTCs, pathologically definable CTCs (PDCTCs), and CAMLs and to analyze PD-L1 expression. In some patients, discordance in PD-L1 expression between tissue and CTCs was observed, suggesting the potential utility of CTCs as predictive tools for therapeutic response. More recently, there have been reports of combining single-cell RNA sequencing with CTCs isolated by CellSieve™ to track intratumoral PD-L1 expression heterogeneity. However, technical limitations persist in CTC-based PD-L1 analysis. Antigen-independent methods carry a risk of false positives due to the potential capture of non-tumor cells (e.g., macrophages, MDSCs), while EpCAM-based approaches may result in false negatives by failing to detect CTCs in the EMT state. Particularly, in cancers with active EMT transition, a single method may not fully capture the immunological characteristics of CTCs. Recent multicenter studies have reported attempts to improve sensitivity by combining EpCAM-based and size-based separation technologies to address these false signal issues, with initial results being evaluated positively. To address these challenges, multiplexed analytical strategies combining CTC isolation with single-cell genomic analysis, RNA sequencing, fluorescence in situ hybridization (FISH), and high-resolution flow cytometry have been proposed. Notably, advances in microfluidic-based technologies now allow for the high-purity isolation of even rare populations of CTCs, enabling precise discrimination among subtypes and detailed immunophenotypic analysis. Recently, studies have also reported the use of CTC-derived organoid models or CTC-xenograft (PDX) models to predict ICI sensitivity ex vivo, suggesting the potential to contribute to therapeutic strategy design beyond simple monitoring. In conclusion, CTC-based PD-L1 analysis is a promising strategy to complement the limitations of tissue biopsy, but it has not yet been established as a standardized clinical assay. Challenges such as low CTC counts, inter-platform result discrepancies, and technical sensitivity issues remain to be addressed. Future efforts should focus on ensuring consistency across platforms, improving sensitivity and specificity, developing optimal separation methods for each tumor type, and analyzing interactions with immune cell populations. Furthermore, the accumulation of multicenter clinical studies and real-world evidence in actual clinical settings will be essential for the formal integration of CTC-based immune markers into ICI response prediction.

7.1.2 Cell-Free DNA (cfDNA), More Specifically, Circulating Tumor DNA (ctDNA)

Alongside CTCs discussed above, ctDNA has become a central analyte in liquid biopsy-based immuno-oncology research. As ctDNA noninvasively reflects tumor-derived genetic information, it is utilized in various aspects such as predicting therapeutic response, disease monitoring, and detecting treatment resistance, with active efforts to apply these approaches to immune checkpoint inhibitor (ICI) therapy. Recent prospective and retrospective cohort studies have repeatedly reported correlations between ctDNA dynamics and ICI response (ORR, PFS, OS), reinforcing its clinical significance as an "early response signal" preceding radiographic changes [7]. Immune checkpoint inhibitors (ICIs) have emerged as a novel therapeutic strategy for various solid tumors, including non-small cell lung cancer (NSCLC), melanoma, and triple-negative breast cancer (TNBC), providing long-term survival benefits for some patients. However, prediction of therapeutic response remains uncertain, and early in treatment, no response (primary resistance) or rapid emergence of resistance after a transient response (acquired resistance) are frequently observed, presenting limitations in actual clinical application. As a strategy to overcome the heterogeneity and unpredictability of therapeutic response, monitoring technologies based on circulating tumor DNA (ctDNA) have recently attracted attention. For example, accumulating reports indicate that early clearance of ctDNA in neoadjuvant chemo-immunotherapy (chemo-IO) for resectable NSCLC is associated with long-term prognosis, and long-term follow-up from the NADIM trial (NCT03081689) has confirmed the survival benefit of immunotherapy, further emphasizing the need for ctDNA biomarker research [8]. In particular, due to the frequent occurrence of pseudoprogression (an immune cell infiltration phenomenon that mimics false-positive disease progression) during ICI therapy, it is difficult to accurately assess therapeutic response early on using conventional imaging alone [7]. In such cases, a rapid decrease in ctDNA levels after initiation of therapy is emerging as a powerful indicator to distinguish true response from nonresponse. Recent studies have reported that changes in ctDNA concentration before and after ICI therapy are closely associated with clinical response [9]. For instance, in patients with advanced melanoma, those in whom ctDNA was undetectable immediately before or within 5 weeks of starting immunotherapy showed significantly improved progression-free survival (PFS) compared to those with persistent ctDNA detection [9]. Similar findings have been observed in various solid tumors, including non-small cell lung cancer (NSCLC), uveal melanoma, and high-frequency MSI colorectal cancer. Notably, the NADIM trial (NCT03081689) demonstrated that early ctDNA clearance after treatment could serve as a more sensitive predictor of therapeutic outcome than radiological response. Beyond quantitative monitoring, ctDNA is also used to predict immunotherapy response through analysis of tumor mutational burden (TMB).

While tissue-based TMB measurement has been standard, blood-based TMB (bTMB) is gaining attention for its noninvasiveness and potential for repeated assessment. Analyses derived from the POPLAR/OAK studies and the prospective exploratory B-F1RST trial (first-line atezolizumab) have reported that bTMB is associated with clinical benefit, and the randomized phase 3 BFAST cohort C suggested that bTMB could assist in treatment selection based on predefined cut-off values [10, 11, 12]. The IMpower110 study showed that higher bTMB in NSCLC patients correlated with better response rates to atezolizumab, indicating that bTMB may play an important role in therapeutic decision-making. However, the precise cut-off values, gene panel composition, and interpretation guidelines for bTMB have yet to be standardized, necessitating further research for clinical application. Currently, representative commercial platforms supporting such analyses include Guardant360® CDx and FoundationOne® Liquid CDx. Both platforms are FDA-approved cfDNA-based companion diagnostics and are used to assess eligibility for immunotherapy. Guardant360® CDx utilizes ctDNA to evaluate microsatellite instability-high (MSI-H) status and is applied as a criterion for pembrolizumab use. In 2021, this platform received FDA approval for ctDNA-based MSI-H detection, providing an important alternative for patients in whom tissue biopsy is not feasible or repeated monitoring is required. MSI-H and mismatch repair deficiency (dMMR) are molecular biomarkers closely associated with ICI response. In 2017, the FDA approved pembrolizumab (Keytruda®) for use across all solid tumors with MSI-H or dMMR status. This marked the first approval of immunotherapy based on a molecular biomarker regardless of tumor origin, representing the advent of tumor-agnostic therapy. The approval was based on an integrated analysis of five clinical trials involving a total of 149 patients, reporting an overall response rate (ORR) of 39.6%, a complete response (CR) of 7.0%, and a partial response (PR) of 32.6% [13]. Among responders, 78% maintained their response for at least 6 months, and 53% survived for more than 1 year [13]. Additionally, FoundationOne® Liquid CDx assesses TMB-high status (≥10 mut/Mb) via ctDNA, and through the Keynote-158 study, the response to pembrolizumab therapy, demonstrating the clinical utility of prediction. Studies have suggested that patients with TMB-high status may exhibit improved objective response rates (ORRs) and disease control rates (DCRs) across various solid tumors. Consequently, in 2020, the FDA approved the use of pembrolizumab based on this testing. ctDNA is also utilized as a tool to elucidate mechanisms of resistance to immunotherapy, with the following examples. Mutations in genes such as STK11, KEAP1, PTEN, JAK1/2, and β-catenin are associated with low responsiveness to immune checkpoint inhibitors (ICIs), and these can be noninvasively identified through cfDNA analysis [14]. In particular, STK11 mutations in NSCLC have been identified as a representative genetic factor inducing poor response to pembrolizumab monotherapy, providing a basis for establishing individualized treatment strategies [14, 15]. In a study involving patients with non-small cell lung cancer, plasma was collected prior to administration of immune checkpoint inhibitors and analyzed using an amplicon-based NGS panel covering 36 genes. As a result, ctDNA mutations were detected in 78% (67 out of 86) of patients, and the following molecular alterations showed a strong correlation with treatment response. Patients harboring PTEN or STK11 mutations were significantly associated with early progressive disease following immunotherapy, interpreted as resistance mutations related to immune evasion mechanisms or defects in antigen presentation. In contrast, transversion mutations in KRAS and TP53 were more frequently observed in responders, suggesting that increased tumor antigenicity and neoantigen load may facilitate a more robust immune response in these patient groups. Most importantly, patients who exhibited a significant reduction in ctDNA levels within a few weeks after initiation of therapy showed a marked extension in both progression-free survival (PFS) and overall survival (OS). This demonstrates that ctDNA is a highly valuable clinical tool, as it can reflect tumor response to treatment more rapidly than radiological changes. A representative prospective clinical trial validating ctDNA-guided therapeutic intervention is the c-TRAK TN trial (NCT03145961) [16]. In this study, patients with triple-negative breast cancer underwent serial monitoring of ctDNA at 3-month intervals following completion of primary therapy (surgery, radiotherapy, adjuvant chemotherapy). Upon detection of increased ctDNA levels, pembrolizumab was administered as an early intervention prior to radiological or clinical recurrence. Patients with confirmed ctDNA elevation were randomized to either the pembrolizumab treatment group or the observation group. The primary endpoint of the study was a reduction in ctDNA concentration, while disease-free survival and overall OS were set as secondary endpoints. This study is significant in that it clinically validated a precision medicine approach that adjusts the timing of therapeutic intervention based on real-time ctDNA dynamics, going beyond simple prognostic prediction. It suggests an expanded role for ctDNA—not merely as a "monitoring marker" of treatment response, but as an actionable indicator that can guide therapeutic intervention. Technically, cfDNA-based MSI detection offers advantages in situations where tissue acquisition is challenging; however, unresolved issues such as low tumor DNA fraction and low allele frequency continue to limit sensitivity. To overcome these technical limitations, advanced methods such as digital PCR, ultrasensitive NGS, and NaME-PrO (nuclease-assisted minor-allele enrichment with probe overlap) are being developed. Recently, studies have also been conducted to predict immunotherapy response by analyzing copy number instability (CNI) in cfDNA [17]. It has been reported that patients with high cfDNA CNI levels across various solid tumors exhibit better responses to immunotherapy, which is biologically linked to increased genomic instability of the tumor, enhancing its recognition by the immune system [18]. In cfDNA-based analyses, clonal hematopoiesis of indeterminate potential (CHIP), as described in the previous chapter, must also be considered as a variable. CHIP, which frequently occurs in elderly patients, involves genes such as TP53, DNMT3A, and ASXL1. It can induce mutations, and if these are mistaken for tumor-derived mutations, it may lead to confusion in treatment strategies. To prevent this, leukocyte-based paired sequencing or algorithm-based filtering techniques should be employed concurrently.

Overall, ctDNA can play a pivotal role throughout the entire process of immunotherapy (prognostic prediction, monitoring of treatment response, detection of resistance, etc.), and is establishing itself as a noninvasive biomarker that complements the limitations of tissue biopsy. In the future, it will be necessary to develop advanced platforms linked to new technologies such as fragmentomics, methylation profiling, and multi-omics integrated analysis. Based on these advancements, large-scale prospective clinical studies will be required to firmly establish ctDNA-based companion diagnostics for immunotherapy.

Based on the current evidence, ctDNA demonstrates potential as a reliable molecular biomarker for early prediction and real-time monitoring of ICI treatment response. In particular, while the prediction of immunotherapy response is limited when relying solely on single biomarkers (such as PD-L1 or tumor mutational burden), ctDNA offers significant advantages by enabling the detection of various gene mutations (e.g., STK11, PTEN, TP53, KEAP1) as well as dynamic changes before and after treatment. Furthermore, as multigene panel analysis technology for plasma cfDNA becomes more sophisticated, ctDNA is evolving into a core platform for multivariate diagnostic algorithms to predict immunotherapy response. For ctDNA-based assessment of immunotherapy response to become a clinical standard, it will be essential to improve the sensitivity and specificity of analytical platforms, establish optimal cut-off values, develop integrated models with co-biomarkers, and, most importantly, demonstrate survival benefits through prospective multicenter clinical trials. Through these efforts, ctDNA can be actively utilized in clinical practice as a key companion diagnostic tool for immunotherapy decision-making.

7.1.3 Proteins and Cytokines Detected in Plasma

Immune-regulatory proteins circulating in the plasma of patients with solid tumors, particularly PD-1 and PD-L1, have shown potential as biomarkers for predicting response to immune checkpoint inhibitor (ICI) therapy. Unlike tissue- or CTC-based analyses, these proteins can be measured noninvasively in plasma, facilitating repeated monitoring and expanding research in this area. For example, Okuma et al. (Clinical Lung Cancer, 2018) quantified plasma PD-L1 levels in patients with advanced NSCLC and reported that those with high pretreatment concentrations exhibited lower response rates to nivolumab [19]. This provides evidence that circulating protein markers can predict immunotherapy response independently of tissue expression.

In particular, soluble PD-1/PD-L1 (sPD-1/sPD-L1), unlike the membranous forms (mPD-1/mPD-L1) expressed on the cell surface, circulate freely in plasma and are known to influence immune responses. These soluble forms bind to receptors on the surface of immune cells, inducing T cell inhibition and thereby reinforcing an immunosuppressive environment. In patients with non-small cell lung cancer (NSCLC), higher pretreatment plasma sPD-L1 levels have been associated with lower response rates to nivolumab, suggesting that sPD-L1 concentrations before and after ICI therapy may serve as prognostic indicators [19]. Weber et al. (Cancer Immunology Research, 2018), in a study of 119 melanoma patients, demonstrated that those with high sPD-L1 levels had shorter progression-free survival (PFS) after nivolumab treatment, further supporting the clinical utility of plasma-based PD-L1 assessment.

Subsequent studies in various solid tumors have also observed that high pre- or on-treatment levels of sPD-1 and sPD-L1 are associated with treatment resistance and lower survival rates. This suggests that elevated circulating sPD-1/PD-L1 concentrations may reduce the efficacy of immune checkpoint blockade, thereby lowering immunotherapy response rates. Lim et al. (Clinical Cancer Research, 2019) demonstrated that patients with metastatic melanoma who had high sPD-L1 concentrations exhibited significantly lower overall survival (OS) compared to those with low concentrations and suggested that changes in sPD-L1 levels during treatment may serve as an important indicator of long-term survival. However, the concentration of these circulating proteins can also increase in non-tumor physiological states such as inflammatory diseases, aging, and pregnancy, making it challenging to establish a universally applicable baseline. In addition, serum protein signatures are being proposed as tools for predicting responses to immune checkpoint inhibitors. Studies tracking changes in serum proteins following anti-PD-1 therapy in patients with metastatic melanoma have reported that specific protein combinations (e.g., CRP, SAA1, β2-microglobulin) are significantly associated with treatment outcomes [20]. Sanmamed et al. (Annals of Oncology, 2017) found that concurrent elevations of CRP and IL-8 in patients with melanoma and NSCLC were associated with lower response rates to immunotherapy and more rapid disease progression, indicating that a panel-based approach may enhance clinical sensitivity and specificity compared to single-protein markers [21]. Cytokines are also being evaluated as important prognostic biomarkers. For example, IL-8 is known to create an immunosuppressive environment and inhibit antitumor immune responses, and several studies have reported that blood levels of IL-8 decrease after treatment in patients who respond well to ICI therapy. In patients with NSCLC and melanoma, such changes have been linked to long-term survival, and combinations of other cytokines such as IL-6, IFN-γ, and TNF-α have also been shown to distinguish responders from nonresponders. Notably, the observation that cytokine profiles change markedly before and after treatment in patients who develop immune-related adverse events (irAEs) suggests that cytokine analysis may be useful not only for predicting treatment response but also for anticipating immune-related toxicities [22]. Thus, analysis of circulating proteins and cytokines can complement the limitations of tissue biopsy and provide practical assistance in predicting and monitoring responses to immunotherapy. However, interpretation of these biomarkers requires caution due to the lack of established cut-off values, variability related to patients' underlying diseases or physiological states, and the inherent complexity of immune responses. Ensuring quantitative consistency across different analytical platforms and establishing normal reference ranges are also essential challenges for clinical application. In conclusion, sPD-1/PD-L1, serum protein signatures, and cytokine panels are all promising blood-based biomarker candidates for predicting prognosis and monitoring immune responses to ICI therapy. In the future, the clinical applicability of these markers is expected to increase through the use of multi-biomarker combinations and artificial intelligence-based pattern analysis algorithms. Indeed, recent integrative analyses have reported that applying multi-protein panels, rather than single proteins, improved predictive accuracy by 20–30%, highlighting a key direction for future research on liquid biopsy-based immune biomarkers.

7.1.4 Extracellular Vesicle

In liquid biopsy, extracellular vesicles (EVs) are emerging as novel biomarkers that can overcome the limitations of tissue biopsy. EVs can be secreted not only by tumor cells but also by immune cells such as T cells, dendritic cells, and macrophages, as well as all cells comprising the tumor microenvironment (TME). They contain proteins, RNA, DNA, and lipids, reflecting the molecular characteristics of their cells of origin. EVs mediate intercellular signaling among immune cells and, in particular, have been reported to play a key role in tumor immune evasion by serving as carriers of immune checkpoint proteins, including PD-L1. In particular, tumor-derived exosomes (TDEs) are of interest because they share not only the genetic and immunological information of the tumor but also mechanisms of immune evasion and have emerged as a useful biomarker for predicting immunotherapy responsiveness. The expression levels of exosomal PD-L1 in the plasma of patients with advanced melanoma were quantified, and it was confirmed that patients with high exosomal PD-L1 expression had significantly lower response rates to anti-PD-1 therapy, as well as shorter progression-free survival (PFS) and overall survival (OS). Exosomal PD-L1 showed a negative correlation with the frequency of PD-1$^+$ CD8$^+$ T cells and was significantly associated with IFN-γ levels, demonstrating its value as a real-time indicator of systemic tumor-induced immunosuppression [23]. Subsequent animal model studies demonstrated that inhibition of exosomal PD-L1 secretion induces systemic antitumor immune responses and immune memory formation, thereby alleviating resistance to immune checkpoint inhibitors [24]. These findings highlight the potential of strategies targeting the inhibition or removal of exosomal PD-L1 to enhance the efficacy of immunotherapy. Additionally, studies have reported that among patients with advanced melanoma treated with ipilimumab, those with higher pretreatment expression of PD-1 and CD28 in tumor-derived exosomes exhibited longer PFS and OS, underscoring the importance of EV-based immune markers as critical tools for dynamic assessment of tumor-immune interactions. Furthermore, exosomes derived from immune cells within the tumor microenvironment (TME) have also been identified as important immune regulators. For example, macrophage-derived exosomes can contain immunosuppressive factors such as PD-L1 or TGF-β, thereby promoting tumor growth and immune evasion. Exosomes derived from dendritic cells or T cells carry miRNAs or proteins involved in antigen presentation and T cell activation (or inhibition), thus participating in complex immune responses. Therefore, EVs have the potential to serve as comprehensive indicators that reflect both the activation and suppression of immune responses, extending beyond simple tumor-derived information. Recent advances in single-particle NTA, high-sensitivity ELISA, and microfluidic chip technologies have enabled both quantitative and qualitative analyses of the immune phenotypes of circulating exosomes.

Research is underway to detect not only PD-L1 but also other immunoregulatory proteins such as LAG-3, TIM-3, and CTLA-4 in exosomes. For instance, a study published in 2022 demonstrated that changes in the size and concentration of PD-L1$^+$ exosomes in NSCLC patients were significantly associated with response to pembrolizumab therapy, and a decrease in exosomes during treatment was suggested as a positive indicator for predicting long-term response [25]. Recently, a new type of EV, termed "blebbisomes," has been defined, which are distinguished from conventional exosomes and microvesicles by their unique biogenesis and functions. Blebbisomes are large EVs formed through the blebbing process of the cell membrane, reaching sizes of several micrometers, and are enriched with multiple immunosuppressive immune checkpoint proteins such as PD-L1, PD-L2, B7-H3, VISTA, PVR, and HLA-E. Blebbisomes have been proposed to not only enhance immune evasion by tumor cells but also serve as novel mediators orchestrating complex interactions between tumors and the immune system. This discovery not only redefines the scope of EV-based biomarkers but also provides new molecular insights into the mechanisms of ICI resistance. Nevertheless, several challenges remain for the clinical application of EV-based biomarkers. First, technologies for accurately tracing the cellular origin of exosomes are still insufficient, and it is difficult to reproducibly analyze the dynamic changes of EVs present in minute quantities within samples. Moreover, the interactions between immune cell-derived and tumor-derived EVs are complex, making interpretation based on a single marker challenging. Despite these challenges, EVs are emerging as a powerful platform for noninvasive assessment of immune dynamics that are difficult to capture through tissue biopsy. In the future, integrating multi-omics analyses of miRNAs, proteins, and surface markers within EVs, combined with AI-based pattern recognition algorithms, may enable the prediction of immunotherapeutic responses and is expected to become a key tool for monitoring.

7.1.5 T-Cell Receptor Repertoire

One of the recently highlighted analytical indicators in the field of immuno-oncology is the T-cell receptor (TCR) repertoire, which refers to the diversity and clonality of T cells possessing different TCRs. Unlike conventional tumor-centric biomarkers such as PD-L1 and TMB, TCR repertoire analysis serves as an immune-centric biomarker that directly reflects the reactivity of the patient's immune system itself. Although traditionally not included within the scope of liquid biopsy, peripheral blood T-cell analysis is emerging as a novel noninvasive biomarker for predicting immunotherapy response and analyzing immune dynamics.

Immune checkpoint inhibitors (ICIs) play a central role in reactivating immune responses against tumors by restoring exhausted cytotoxic T cells and inhibiting the immunosuppressive function of regulatory T cells (Tregs). Accordingly, various studies are underway to evaluate the distribution, phenotype, and clonality of T cells in peripheral blood to predict therapeutic response, serving as a complementary approach to tissue biopsy. Among the recently highlighted analytical indicators in immuno-oncology is the T-cell receptor (TCR) repertoire, which refers to the diversity and clonality of T cells with different TCRs. TCR repertoire analysis, unlike conventional tumor-centric biomarkers such as PD-L1 and TMB, can directly reflect the reactivity of the patient's immune system as an immune-centric biomarker. Although not traditionally included in the category of liquid biopsy, peripheral blood T-cell analysis is emerging as a novel noninvasive biomarker for predicting immunotherapy response and analyzing immune dynamics.

Immune checkpoint inhibitors (ICIs) play a central role in reactivating immune responses against tumors by restoring exhausted cytotoxic T cells and inhibiting the immunosuppressive function of regulatory T cells (Tregs). Therefore, various studies are being conducted to evaluate the distribution, phenotype, and clonality of T cells in peripheral blood to predict therapeutic response, and this approach is gaining attention as a complement to tissue biopsy. High TCR diversity or clonal expansion of specific clones has been associated with response to ICI therapy, and in particular, high diversity before treatment and expansion of specific antigen-specific clones after treatment are linked to a favorable prognosis.

T cells can be readily isolated from a patient's peripheral blood using density gradient centrifugation and selective separation of CD4+/CD8+ cells (flow cytometry), after which TCR repertoire analysis can be performed to determine correlations with therapeutic response [26]. The TCR consists of α and β chains, with the CDR3 (complementarity-determining region 3) of the β chain being a key structure formed through V(D) J gene recombination that determines the antigen specificity of the T cell. The diversity of CDR3 sequences and the degree of clonal expansion are directly associated with the strength of T-cell responses to tumor antigens.

Clinically, changes in the diversity and clonality of the TCR repertoire have been shown in various studies to be closely linked to ICI treatment response. In a study of patients with renal cell carcinoma treated with nivolumab, there was little difference in TCR diversity among patients before treatment, but marked clonal expansion was observed in responders 1 month after treatment, which persisted throughout the treatment period. In patients with metastatic melanoma, expansion of new TCR clones was observed in those receiving a combination of personalized neoantigen vaccine and ICI therapy, which was associated with long-term memory T-cell responses and survival benefits [27].

In a study of NSCLC patients, pretreatment TCR clonality was not directly associated with overall survival (OS), but a decrease in TCR diversity was significantly linked to reduced survival, and a decrease in TCR convergence, which indicates the degree of convergence toward specific antigen specificity, was paradoxically associated with better prognosis. Furthermore, by linking patterns of T-cell infiltration in tumor tissue with peripheral TCR dynamics, high TCR diversity and immune activation signatures have been reported to increase the response rate to PD-1 inhibitors [28].

The expression of PD-1$^+$ T cells in the blood is also evaluated as an important indicator. In patients with melanoma and renal cell carcinoma, PD-1$^+$ lymphocytes in peripheral blood correspond to tumor-specific neoantigen-recognizing T cells, and their presence is associated with therapeutic responsiveness to agents such as pembrolizumab. In this context, functional expansion analysis of these T cells (MANAFEST assay) has been proposed as a platform capable of sensitively tracking antitumor immune responses [29].

Of particular note is TCR convergence, a phenomenon in which multiple TCR clones with structurally similar sequences converge in response to a specific antigen. In melanoma patients, those with high TCR convergence demonstrated higher response rates to anti-PD-1 therapy, suggesting that this may serve as an indirect indicator of shared antigen specificity [30].

Collectively, TCR repertoire analysis is rapidly establishing itself as a next-generation immune biomarker for predicting and monitoring responses to immuno-oncology therapies. In the future, it is expected that integrated indicators such as TCR diversity, convergence, and clonal expansion will enable the development of personalized immunotherapy strategies for individual patients.

Moreover, with technological advances and the advent of multilayered analyses, liquid biopsy-based biomarkers for predicting immunotherapy responsiveness are showing increasingly clear directionality and differentiation. Among these, cfDNA/ctDNA currently represents the platform closest to clinical application, providing some of the few examples that have been commercialized as companion diagnostics through quantitative analysis, plasma-based TMB assessment (bTMB), and MSI-H diagnosis, all of which have received FDA approval. The ability to serially track molecular changes in tumors through repeated blood sampling also enhances its practicality, and to date, it has become the most widely utilized foundational platform.

Although TCR repertoire and T-cell convergence analyses remain in the early stages of clinical implementation, they are regarded as highly promising biomarkers due to their high-precision, antigen-specific analytical capabilities. Clonal expansion, reduced diversity, and degree of convergence are increasingly being validated as robust indicators for predicting therapeutic response and survival and are likely to evolve into next-generation core tools for precision prediction in immunotherapy.

Circulating tumor cells (CTCs) are significant in that they provide information difficult to obtain from tissue biopsies, such as cell-level phenotypic analysis, elucidation of EMT status, and assessment of PD-L1 expression. However, their extremely low concentration in blood, limitations due to epithelial dependence (EpCAM-based detection), and the highly heterogeneous nature of these cell populations result in instability in sensitivity and specificity, thus limiting their clinical application.

Extracellular vesicles (EVs), particularly exosomal PD-L1, support molecular mechanisms that can explain both responsiveness and resistance to immune checkpoint inhibitors. Recently, the definition of new EV subtypes, such as blebbisomes, has expanded the scope of EV research. Analyses of tumor-immune interactions via various immune cell-derived EVs are also increasing; however, challenges such as their minute abundance, lack of standardized analytical methods, and difficulties in tracing their origin remain significant barriers to commercialization.

Protein- and cytokine-based biomarkers offer the advantages of relatively easy accessibility and well-established analytical technologies. However, their variability is high due to various background factors such as inflammation, infection, aging, and physiological conditions, making it difficult to ensure clinical reliability with a single indicator. Therefore, approaches based on multiplex protein signatures or integrated use with other analytes are being proposed as more desirable strategies.

In summary, cfDNA-based analyses are currently the most advanced in terms of technological and clinical maturity and are directly utilized in therapeutic decision-making. In contrast, TCR repertoire analysis is distinguished by its ability to precisely reflect the qualitative aspects of immune responses. There is significant potential for expansion as a next-generation core biomarker. The remaining platforms (CTC, EV, proteins/cytokines) may serve as complementary approaches in specific contexts, and in the future, the integration of all these through multi-omic integration strategies is expected to dramatically enhance diagnostic and predictive accuracy. This demonstrates that liquid biopsy can evolve beyond a simple auxiliary tool to become a central pillar reshaping the therapeutic paradigm in the era of immuno-oncology.

References

1. Reck M, Rodríguez-Abreu D, Robinson AG, Hui R, Csőszi T, Fülöp A, et al. Pembrolizumab versus chemotherapy for PD-L1–positive non–small-cell lung cancer. N Engl J Med. Massachusetts Medical Society. 2016 [cited 2025 Sep 4]. Available from: https://www.nejm.org/doi/full/10.1056/NEJMoa1606774.
2. Reck M, Rodríguez-Abreu D, Robinson AG, Hui R, Csőszi T, Fülöp A, et al. Five-year outcomes with pembrolizumab versus chemotherapy for metastatic non-small-cell lung cancer with PD-L1 tumor proportion score ≥ 50. J Clin Oncol. 2021;39(21):2339–49.
3. Gandhi L, Rodríguez-Abreu D, Gadgeel S, Esteban E, Felip E, Angelis FD, et al. Pembrolizumab plus chemotherapy in metastatic non–small-cell lung cancer. N Engl J Med [Internet]. 2018 [cited 2025 Sep 4]. Available from: https://www.nejm.org/doi/full/10.1056/NEJMoa1801005.
4. Ilie M, Long-Mira E, Bence C, Butori C, Lassalle S, Bouhlel L, et al. Comparative study of the PD-L1 status between surgically resected specimens and matched biopsies of NSCLC patients reveal major discordances: a potential issue for anti-PD-L1 therapeutic strategies. Ann Oncol. 2016;27(1):147–53.
5. Nicolazzo C, Raimondi C, Mancini M, Caponnetto S, Gradilone A, Gandini O, et al. Monitoring PD-L1 positive circulating tumor cells in non-small cell lung cancer patients treated with the PD-1 inhibitor Nivolumab. Sci Rep. 2016;6(1):31726.
6. Adams DL, Adams DK, Alpaugh RK, Cristofanilli M, Martin SS, Chumsri S, et al. Circulating cancer-associated macrophage-like cells differentiate malignant breast cancer and benign breast conditions. Cancer Epidemiol Biomarkers Prev. 2016;25(7):1037–42.
7. Cabel L, Proudhon C, Romano E, Girard N, Lantz O, Stern MH, et al. Clinical potential of circulating tumour DNA in patients receiving anticancer immunotherapy. Nat Rev Clin Oncol. 2018;15(10):639–50.

8. Provencio M, Nadal E, Insa A, Campelo RG, Casal J, Dómine M, et al. Perioperative chemotherapy and nivolumab in non-small-cell lung cancer (NADIM): 5-year clinical outcomes from a multicentre, single-arm, phase 2 trial. Lancet Oncol. 2024;25(11):1453–64.
9. Cabel L, Riva F, Servois V, Livartowski A, Daniel C, Rampanou A, et al. Circulating tumor DNA changes for early monitoring of anti-PD1 immunotherapy: a proof-of-concept study. Ann Oncol. 2017;28(8):1996–2001.
10. Gandara DR, Paul SM, Kowanetz M, Schleifman E, Zou W, Li Y, et al. Blood-based tumor mutational burden as a predictor of clinical benefit in non-small-cell lung cancer patients treated with atezolizumab. Nat Med. 2018;24(9):1441–8.
11. Kim ES, Velcheti V, Mekhail T, Yun C, Shagan SM, Hu S, et al. Blood-based tumor mutational burden as a biomarker for atezolizumab in non-small cell lung cancer: the phase 2 B-F1RST trial. Nat Med. 2022;28(5):939.
12. Peters S, Dziadziuszko R, Morabito A, Felip E, Gadgeel SM, Cheema P, et al. Atezolizumab versus chemotherapy in advanced or metastatic NSCLC with high blood-based tumor mutational burden: primary analysis of BFAST cohort C randomized phase 3 trial. Nat Med. 2022;28(9):1831–9.
13. Le DT, Uram JN, Wang H, Bartlett BR, Kemberling H, Eyring AD, et al. PD-1 blockade in tumors with mismatch-repair deficiency. N Engl J Med. 2015;372(26):2509–20.
14. Jure-Kunkel M, Wu S, Xiao F, Abdullah SE, Gao G, Englert JM, et al. Somatic STK11/LKB1 mutations to confer resistance to immune checkpoint inhibitors as monotherapy or in combination in advanced NSCLC. J Clin Oncol. 2018;36(15_suppl):3028.
15. Skoulidis F, Araujo HA, Do MT, Qian Y, Sun X, Galan-Cobo A, et al. CTLA4 blockade abrogates KEAP1/STK11-related resistance to PD-(L)1 inhibitors. Nature. 2024;635(8038):462–71.
16. Turner NC, Swift C, Jenkins B, Kilburn L, Coakley M, Beaney M, et al. Results of the c-TRAK TN trial: a clinical trial utilising ctDNA mutation tracking to detect molecular residual disease and trigger intervention in patients with moderate- and high-risk early-stage triple-negative breast cancer. Ann Oncol. 2023;34(2):200–11.
17. Jensen TJ, Goodman AM, Kato S, Ellison CK, Daniels GA, Kim L, et al. Genome-wide sequencing of cell-free DNA identifies copy-number alterations that can be used for monitoring response to immunotherapy in cancer patients. Mol Cancer Ther. 2019;18(2):448–58.
18. Weiss GJ, Beck J, Braun DP, Bornemann-Kolatzki K, Barilla H, Cubello R, et al. Tumor cell-free DNA copy number instability predicts therapeutic response to immunotherapy. Clin Cancer Res. 2017;23(17):5074–81.
19. Okuma Y, Wakui H, Utsumi H, Sagawa Y, Hosomi Y, Kuwano K, et al. Soluble programmed cell death ligand 1 as a novel biomarker for nivolumab therapy for non–small-cell lung cancer. Clin Lung Cancer. 2018;19(5):410–7.e1.
20. Weber JS, Sznol M, Sullivan RJ, Blackmon S, Boland G, Kluger HM, et al. A serum protein signature associated with outcome after anti-PD-1 therapy in metastatic melanoma. Cancer Immunol Res. 2018;6(1):79–86.
21. Sanmamed MF, Perez-Gracia JL, Schalper KA, Fusco JP, Gonzalez A, Rodriguez-Ruiz ME, et al. Changes in serum interleukin-8 (IL-8) levels reflect and predict response to anti-PD-1 treatment in melanoma and non-small-cell lung cancer patients. Ann Oncol. 2017;28(8):1988–95.
22. Lim SY, Lee JH, Gide TN, Menzies AM, Guminski A, Carlino MS, et al. Circulating cytokines predict immune-related toxicity in melanoma patients receiving anti-PD-1–based immunotherapy. Clin Cancer Res. 2019;25(5):1557–63.
23. Chen G, Huang AC, Zhang W, Zhang G, Wu M, Xu W, et al. Exosomal PD-L1 contributes to immunosuppression and is associated with anti-PD-1 response. Nature. 2018;560(7718):382–6.
24. Poggio M, Hu T, Pai CC, Chu B, Belair CD, Chang A, et al. Suppression of exosomal PD-L1 induces systemic anti-tumor immunity and memory. Cell. 2019;177(2):414–27.e13.
25. Wang Y, Niu X, Cheng Y, Zhang Y, Xia L, Xia W, et al. Exosomal PD-L1 predicts response with immunotherapy in NSCLC patients. Clin Exp Immunol. 2022;208(3):316–22.
26. Rosati E, Dowds CM, Liaskou E, Henriksen EKK, Karlsen TH, Franke A. Overview of methodologies for T-cell receptor repertoire analysis. BMC Biotechnol. 2017;17(1):61.
27. Ott PA, Hu Z, Keskin DB, Shukla SA, Sun J, Bozym DJ, et al. An immunogenic personal neoantigen vaccine for patients with melanoma. Nature. 2017;547(7662):217–21.
28. Giraldo NA, Becht E, Vano Y, Petitprez F, Lacroix L, Validire P, et al. Tumor-infiltrating and peripheral blood T-cell immunophenotypes predict early relapse in localized clear cell renal cell carcinoma. Clin Cancer Res. 2017;23(15):4416–28.
29. Danilova L, Anagnostou V, Caushi JX, Sidhom JW, Guo H, Chan HY, et al. The mutation-associated neoantigen functional expansion of specific T cells (MANAFEST) assay: a sensitive platform for monitoring antitumor immunity. Cancer Immunol Res. 2018;6(8):888–99.
30. Hogan SA, Courtier A, Cheng PF, Jaberg-Bentele NF, Goldinger SM, Manuel M, et al. Peripheral blood TCR repertoire profiling may facilitate patient stratification for immunotherapy against melanoma. Cancer Immunol Res. 2019;7(1):77–85.

Suggested Reading

Pantel K, Alix-Panabières C. Liquid biopsy and minimal residual disease – latest advances and implications for cure. Nat Rev Clin Oncol. 2019;16(7):409–24.

Leighl NB, Page RD, Raymond VM, Daniel DB, Divers SG, Reckamp KL, et al. Clinical utility of comprehensive cell-free DNA analysis to identify genomic biomarkers in patients with newly diagnosed metastatic non-small cell lung cancer. Clin Cancer Res. 2019;25(15):4691–700.

Razavi P, Li BT, Brown DN, Jung B, Hubbell E, Shen R, et al. High-intensity sequencing reveals the sources of plasma circulating cell-free DNA variants. Nat Med. 2019;25(12):1928–37.

Hofman P, Heeke S, Alix-Panabières C, Pantel K. Liquid biopsy in the era of immuno-oncology: is it ready for prime-time use for cancer patients? Ann Oncol. 2019;30(9):1448–59.

Pantel K, Alix-Panabières C. Minimal residual disease as a target for liquid biopsy in patients with solid tumours. Nat Rev Clin Oncol. 2025;22(1):65–77.

Sinoquet L, Jacot W, Quantin X, Alix-Panabières C. Liquid biopsy and immuno-oncology for advanced nonsmall cell lung cancer. Clin Chem. 2023;69(1):23–40.

Mayrhofer M, De Laere B, Whitington T, Van Oyen P, Ghysel C, Ampe J, et al. Cell-free DNA profiling of metastatic prostate cancer reveals microsatellite instability, structural rearrangements and clonal hematopoiesis. Genome Med. 2018;10(1):85.

Shiller M, Johnson M, Auber R, Patel SP. Clinical perspectives on the value of testing for STK11 and KEAP1 mutations in advanced NSCLC. Front Oncol. 2024;14:1459737.

Xi J, Ma CX, O'Shaughnessy J. Current clinical utility of circulating tumor DNA testing in breast cancer: a practical approach. JCO Oncol Pract [Internet]. 2024 [cited 2025 Sep 4]. Available from: https://ascopubs.org/doi/10.1200/OP.24.00274.

Whiteside TL. The potential of tumor-derived exosomes for noninvasive cancer monitoring: an update. Expert Rev Mol Diagn. 2018;18(12):1029–40.

Gibney GT, Weiner LM, Atkins MB. Predictive biomarkers for checkpoint inhibitor-based immunotherapy. Lancet Oncol. 2016;17(12):e542–51.

Anagnostou V, Smith KN, Forde PM, Niknafs N, Bhattacharya R, White J, et al. Evolution of neoantigen landscape during immune checkpoint blockade in non-small cell lung cancer. Cancer Discov. 2017;7(3):264–76.

Gros A, Parkhurst MR, Tran E, Pasetto A, Robbins PF, Ilyas S, et al. Prospective identification of neoantigen-specific lymphocytes in the peripheral blood of melanoma patients. Nat Med. 2016;22(4):433–8.

8 Conclusions and Future Directions

Liquid biopsy is an innovative technology capable of noninvasively reflecting the inherent complexity of cancer, including its spatial and temporal heterogeneity. It has established itself as a core pillar of modern precision medicine and precision oncology. Over the past decade, various prospective and retrospective clinical studies have gradually demonstrated its clinical validity and utility. This trend indicates that liquid biopsy is emerging not merely as a complementary tool to traditional tissue biopsy, but as the "Third Wave" that is transforming the very paradigm of cancer diagnosis and treatment [1].

Currently, the most actively utilized analyte in clinical practice is ctDNA. ctDNA has already received FDA approval for companion diagnostics through quantitative mutation analysis, plasma-based TMB assessment (bTMB), and high-frequency microsatellite instability (MSI-H) detection, and in some areas, clinical trials for early diagnosis have begun. However, several challenges remain in applying these tests to real-world patient populations. In certain cancer types, the sensitivity and specificity of ctDNA-based assays are insufficient, and discrepancies with tissue-based genetic analyses are frequently reported [2]. Particularly in key precision medicine applications such as early cancer detection, minimal residual disease (MRD) monitoring, and assessment of therapeutic response and resistance, sufficient clinical evidence has yet to be accumulated, and both analytical and interpretive improvements are urgently needed [3, 4].

In addition to ctDNA, other analytes such as CTCs, EVs, circulating proteins, immune-related cytokines, and TCR repertoires each possess unique biological advantages, yet their adoption as clinical standards remains limited [5]. This is not solely due to technical immaturity, but also to a combination of factors including variability in sample processing, uncertainty in analytical sensitivity and specificity, complexity in data interpretation, and lack of standardization for pre-analytical variables. In other words, while liquid biopsy has already demonstrated considerable potential, significant technical, biological, and interpretive challenges must still be overcome to translate this potential into reliable clinical utility [6].

In this context, this chapter presents seven key challenges that must be addressed for liquid biopsy to become a routine diagnostic tool in precision medicine. These challenges extend beyond simple technological improvements to include refinement of biological understanding, regulatory validation of analytical methods, large-scale multicenter clinical validation, and integration with clinical workflows. Therefore, the seven items presented here represent shared tasks that must be tackled collaboratively by researchers, clinicians, regulatory agencies, and industry stakeholders in the field of liquid biopsy (Fig. 8.1).

S. I. Kim, Y. Kim, *Liquid Biopsy for Cancer*, https://doi.org/10.1007/978-981-99-4418-7_8

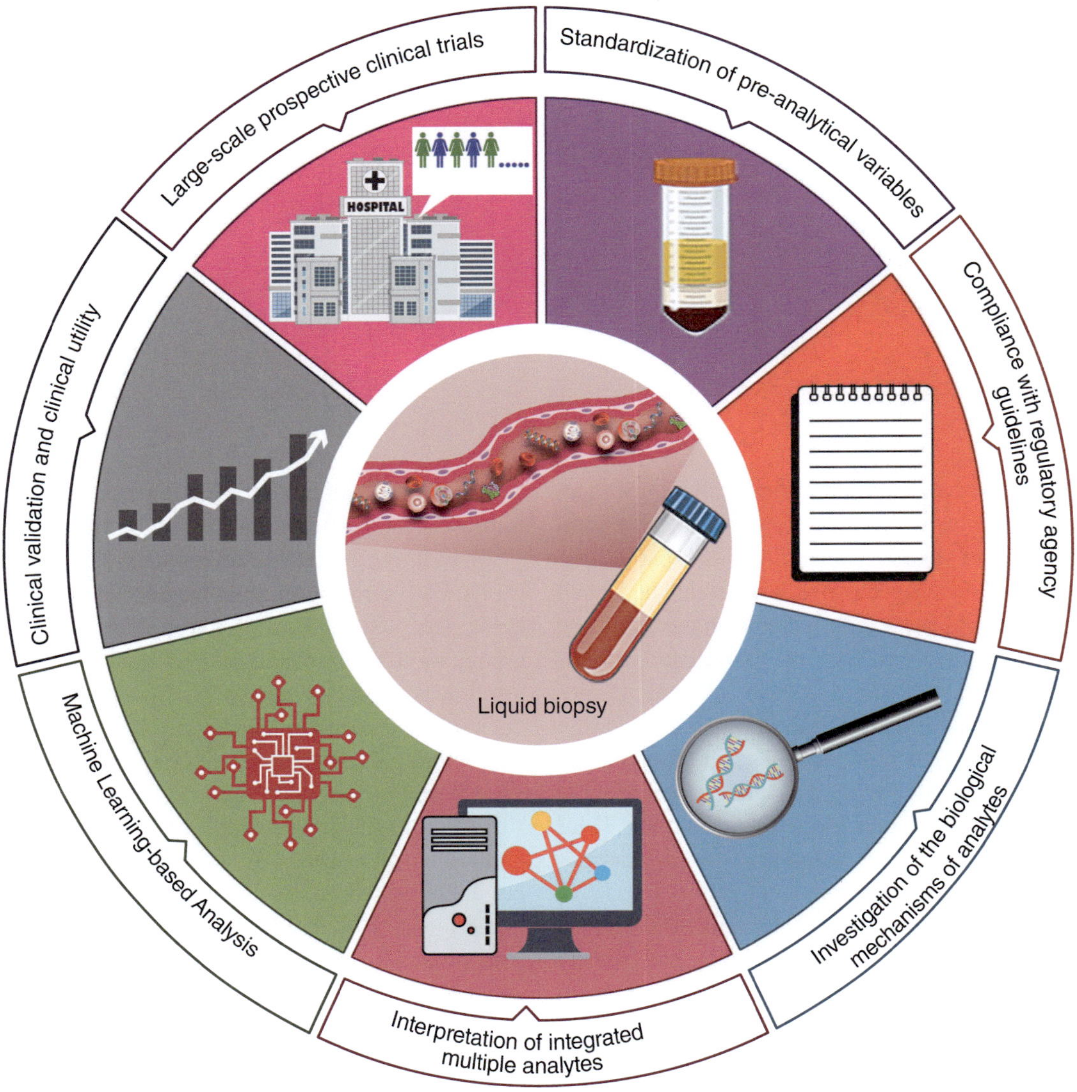

Fig. 8.1 Seven key challenges for implementing liquid biopsy in clinical settings

8.1 Standardization of Pre-Analytical Variables

To ensure the clinical reproducibility and analytical reliability of liquid biopsy, thorough standardization of pre-analytical variables is essential [7]. This includes a series of factors such as sample collection containers, storage temperature and duration, centrifugation conditions, and plasma separation procedures. The processing workflow directly affects the stability and quality of analytes such as cfDNA and EVs, serving as a critical determinant of the sensitivity and specificity of analytical results. Standardization of pre-analytical procedures not only ensures consistency in analysis but also enables comparison and integration across different studies, thereby facilitating the broader adoption of liquid biopsy. In practice, the clinical efficacy demonstrated under controlled conditions in numerous clinical studies often falls short of expectations in real-world clinical settings. This discrepancy is likely due to variability in analytical results stemming from the failure to establish pre-analytical factors, which can ultimately lead to errors in clinical interpretation. Therefore, standardizing pre-analytical variables is a key task that enhances the value of liquid biopsy results and enables comparison and combination of findings across studies, thereby accelerating clinical implementation. Internationally, large-scale consortium efforts are actively underway to address these issues. The EU's SPIDIA4P project aims to standardize the pre-analytical processing of various human specimens, including blood and tissue, and has contributed to the development of CEN/ISO guidelines for in vitro diagnostics, including liquid biopsy [8]. The CANCER-ID consortium, established under the leadership of the Innovative Medicines Initiative (IMI), is validating the standardization and clinical applicability of multiple analytes, including CTCs, cfDNA, and EVs, with a particular focus on enabling inter-institutional data comparability. In the United States, the BloodPAC consortium is centered on ctDNA-based liquid biopsy, laying the groundwork for clinical implementation through assay validation, establishment of reference standards, and the construction of a large-scale data-sharing platform. International collaborative models such as SPIDIA4P, CANCER-ID, and BloodPAC offer concrete solutions to minimize variability in the pre-analytical phase of liquid biopsy and to ensure clinical reliability. Moving forward, these global standardization efforts must be reflected in diagnostic device development, regulatory approval, and clinical trial design, thereby establishing liquid biopsy as a routine tool in precision medicine.

8.2 The Need for Large-Scale Prospective Clinical Trials

For the clinical adoption of liquid biopsy, large-scale, multicenter, prospective clinical trials are essential [9]. While accumulated studies to date have provided important insights into the genetic evolution and molecular dynamics of tumors, most have been limited to small cohorts, single institutions, or retrospective analyses, presenting fundamental limitations for extrapolation to real-world patient care. In high-stakes clinical areas such as companion diagnostics, treatment response monitoring, minimal residual disease (MRD) detection, and early screening, prospective studies with statistically sufficient sample sizes and clearly predefined endpoints are required.

For example, in the IMvigor010 study (evaluating atezolizumab as adjuvant therapy), clinical benefit from immunotherapy was observed only in ctDNA-positive patients, prospectively demonstrating that ctDNA can serve as a criterion for therapeutic intervention. Similarly, the NADIM trial in NSCLC patients showed that those who experienced early clearance of ctDNA during combined immunotherapy and chemotherapy had long-term survival benefits, preceding radiological assessment. These findings establish that ctDNA monitoring is not merely an auxiliary marker but an actionable biomarker capable of guiding therapeutic decisions. However, most studies to date have involved fewer than 100 participants, which is insufficient to establish universal evidence.

In particular, for liquid biopsy studies aimed at screening, clinical trial design must account for disease prevalence. Sensitivity and specificity alone are insufficient to fully evaluate diagnostic performance, as positive predictive value (PPV) and negative predictive value (NPV) vary significantly with prevalence. For instance, the CCGA (Circulating Cell-free Genome Atlas) study, a representative investigation of the Multi-Cancer Early Detection (MCED) platform, enrolled over 15,000 participants to reflect cancer prevalence in real-world clinical scenarios, and as a result, it was possible to precisely calculate not only the sensitivity and specificity of early diagnosis, but also the positive predictive value (PPV) [10]. Conversely, sensitivity and specificity results derived from small-scale cohorts may lead to an increase in false positives and the risk of overtreatment when applied to the general population. Therefore, for screening purposes, liquid biopsy must be comprehensively evaluated using large-scale cohorts and long-term follow-up, assessing not only sensitivity and specificity but also PPV, NPV, concordance rate, and various other clinical performance indicators. This goes beyond merely demonstrating the technical feasibility of the method and constitutes the minimum requirement for verifying its actual clinical utility. Ultimately, for liquid biopsy to become a routine tool in precision medicine beyond the research laboratory, its effectiveness for each cancer type and intended use must be systematically validated through large-scale prospective clinical trials. This is not simply a scientific validation process, but an essential step for liquid biopsy to be trusted as a clinical decision-making tool.

8.3 Verification of Applicability Within the Clinical Workflow

No matter how high the sensitivity and specificity of liquid biopsy technology, it cannot be implemented in clinical practice unless the intended use within the clinical context is clearly defined and its clinical utility is demonstrated. Beyond analytical and clinical validity, liquid biopsy must prove that it can induce meaningful changes in patient treatment decisions and outcomes in order to establish clinical significance. A representative example is cfDNA-based companion diagnostics. The cobas® EGFR Mutation Test v2, targeting EGFR mutations, demonstrated through large-scale prospective studies that administration of EGFR-TKIs such as gefitinib, erlotinib, and osimertinib is effective in patients with mutations detected in plasma cfDNA, leading to FDA approval. However, in practice, there are cases where actionable mutations are detected in plasma cfDNA but not confirmed in tumor tissue. In such situations, if treatment is prescribed based solely on cfDNA analysis, there must be scientific evidence to support whether patients actually gain a survival benefit or are exposed to unnecessary toxicity. Therefore, beyond simply detecting mutations, study designs are needed to verify whether treatment strategies based on blood-based analysis actually improve OS and PFS in patients. Furthermore, in applications such as MRD (minimal residual disease) monitoring and assessment of treatment response, empirical evidence is required to demonstrate how much earlier liquid biopsy can detect disease compared to conventional imaging, and how quickly and accurately it can guide clinical decision-making [11]. For example, in the IMvigor010 clinical trial, adjuvant atezolizumab showed significant efficacy only in urothelial carcinoma patients who were ctDNA-positive after curative resection. This indicates that ctDNA monitoring can serve as a pivotal point for therapeutic intervention, rather than merely an auxiliary marker. In breast cancer, the c-TRAK-TN study monitored postsurgical ctDNA in triple-negative breast cancer patients through serial sampling, enabling early detection of molecular recurrence before radiological relapse and suggesting the potential for immunotherapy intervention. Another advantage of integrating liquid biopsy into the actual workflow is its ability to complement the limitations of imaging assessments. In breast cancer patients with frequent bone metastases, it is difficult to quantify disease activity using conventional imaging alone. In contrast, changes in ctDNA concentration or the emergence of specific mutations can sensitively reflect molecular changes not captured by imaging, serving as early indicators of treatment resistance. In this way, liquid biopsy plays a complementary role to radiological findings and is likely to become a central component of multimodal monitoring strategies in the long term. Of course, liquid biopsy cannot completely replace radiological diagnosis. However, the integrated use of liquid biopsy and imaging throughout the processes of diagnosis, treatment, and follow-up can enhance clinical workflow efficiency and is increasingly being proposed as a strategy to maximize integration [12]. To achieve this, large-scale, well-controlled, and well-designed prospective cohort studies must be conducted in parallel, based on liquid biopsy technologies with proven analytical reliability and clinical validity. Ultimately, technical excellence alone is insufficient for successful integration into clinical workflows. There must be a clear definition of which patient populations, at what time points, and for what clinical purposes the technology will be applied, and corresponding clinical evidence must be established. Only through such a multilayered validation process can liquid biopsy truly become a patient-centered precision medicine tool.

8.4 Integrated Analysis of Multiple Analytes

To date, most reported liquid biopsy studies have focused on single-analyte approaches, and these single-analyte strategies commonly reveal limitations in analytical sensitivity, interpretive accuracy, and representation of biological diversity. For example, while ctDNA can reflect certain aspects of the tumor genome, it does not capture functional changes at the transcriptome or protein level. CTCs offer the advantage of providing precise information at the cellular level, but their extremely low detection rates and analytical complexity pose significant challenges. EVs stably contain various biomolecules, but difficulties remain in standardizing isolation and determining tumor origin. To overcome the structural limitations of single-analyte strategies, integrated multi-analyte analysis approaches have recently been actively pursued. Methods that analyze ctDNA mutation data together with EV-derived miRNAs, CTC phenotypic information, cfDNA methylation patterns, and circulating protein or metabolite data can more precisely reflect the complex biological characteristics of tumors. For instance, the CancerSEEK study, which combined cfDNA-based methylation signatures with protein panels, achieved higher sensitivity and specificity than single-marker approaches, and a large-scale, multicenter prospective clinical trial (involving 10,000 participants) demonstrated the potential for early detection of specific cancer types [13]. Additionally, Grail's Galleri platform, which integrates cfDNA methylation patterns with machine learning algorithms, has been applied to multi-cancer early detection (MCED) and is currently being validated for clinical workflow applicability through the SUMMIT and PATHFINDER studies. Another example is a study integrating EV-derived protein signatures with ctDNA mutation dynamics, which reported a significant improvement in recurrence prediction sensitivity compared to the use of individual analytes alone. Such multi-analyte strategies are particularly advantageous for capturing the complex changes in the tumor microenvironment and have demonstrated superior performance over single biomarkers in predicting immunotherapy response. In particular, when different analytes present in a single blood sample are analyzed in a multivariate manner, not only can diagnostic accuracy be improved, but the scope of application for prognosis prediction and treatment response monitoring can also be greatly expanded. For example, integrating ctDNA mutation burden, EV protein panels, and plasma cytokine signatures enables earlier detection of recurrence before it becomes radiologically apparent, and several studies have reported a 20–30% improvement in early detection rates compared to single-analyte approaches. However, there remains uncertainty as to whether integrated multi-analyte analysis can serve as a fundamental solution. Because each analyte differs in biological origin, release mechanisms, analytical platform sensitivity and specificity, and data interpretation methodologies, simple parallel integration is insufficient. To achieve effective and robust integrated analysis, (1) quantitative compatibility between analytical technologies, (2) standardization of interpretive algorithms and cut-offs, and (3) large-scale, multicenter validation studies demonstrating clinical utility.

Recently, there has been a growing effort to overcome these limitations by combining multi-omics approaches with artificial intelligence (AI)-based machine learning models. AI models that integrate high-dimensional data can identify complex patterns that are undetectable by single-analyte analyses, thereby improving diagnostic accuracy and enabling patient-specific therapeutic predictions. For example, a machine learning model integrating cfDNA methylation profiles, EV miRNA signatures, and serum proteins has been reported to improve the AUC by more than 0.10 compared to single-analyte models in early lung cancer diagnosis.

Ultimately, multi-analyte-based approaches represent a highly promising strategy to address the structural limitations of single-analyte assays.

However, for clinical implementation, multiple barriers must be overcome, including technical complexity, cost burden, data standardization, and regulatory approval processes. Future research should move beyond simple parallel combinations and demonstrate clinical validity and feasibility through integrative designs that reflect underlying biological mechanisms [14]. This will require large-scale, prospective studies supported by international consortia.

8.5 Integration of High-Dimensional Data and Machine Learning-Based Interpretation

The aforementioned multi-analyte integration strategies inevitably generate vast amounts of biological data. Since each analyte differs in origin, unit, and interpretation method, simple parallel comparisons are insufficient. A sophisticated interpretive framework enabling high-dimensional integration is required. In this context, machine learning and AI-based algorithms are emerging as next-generation tools for interpreting liquid biopsy data.

In clinical radiology and pathology, AI-based decision support systems have already demonstrated significant improvements in diagnostic sensitivity and specificity. For instance, combining deep learning models with radiologists' interpretations in mammography or pulmonary nodule detection has resulted in higher accuracy compared to independent readings. These experiences suggest that AI can also make substantial contributions to the precise interpretation of atypical biological signals.

Liquid biopsy likewise involves the complexity of simultaneously considering genomic, transcriptomic, proteomic, and metabolomic data. For example, cfDNA mutations and methylation profiles, fragmentomics, CTC phenotypes, and combinations of EV proteins and miRNAs each provide distinct layers of information. AI-based multivariate models can integratively learn from these data, extracting nonlinear interactions and subtle signal patterns that conventional linear analyses may miss. This not only enhances diagnostic accuracy but also improves prognostic prediction.

A representative example is the CancerSEEK platform, a multi-biomarker-based early cancer detection prototype, which demonstrated its potential in large-scale clinical trials such as the DETECT-A trial. However, due to challenges in managing false positives and integrating into clinical workflows, the platform evolved into CancerGuard, which incorporates cfDNA-based methylation and fragmentomics analyses with machine learning models, resulting in improved sensitivity and specificity. Currently, multicenter prospective validation studies are underway. Thus, AI serves as a core technology enabling the interpretation of multi-analyte liquid biopsy data, offering superior performance compared to single biomarker approaches. Nevertheless, the reported improvements in clinical performance vary 5–20% across studies, and it is more appropriate to emphasize that "clinical accuracy is meaningfully improved" rather than generalizing specific figures.

Ultimately, the interpretation of liquid biopsy data is advancing beyond merely detecting the presence of biomarkers, toward quantitatively modeling the molecular evolution of disease, immune evasion mechanisms, and the dynamics of therapeutic response and resistance. Successful implementation will require multidisciplinary research spanning molecular biology, oncology, statistics, and computer science, as well as the establishment of explainable AI models tailored for clinical application. Only on this foundation can liquid biopsy become a core tool in precision medicine, translating high-dimensional data into clinical decision-making.

8.6 Investigation of the Biological Mechanisms of Analytes

For liquid biopsy to be established as a technology that enables precision medicine, it is essential to secure biological plausibility by demonstrating that the analytes are indeed derived from malignant tumors. While tissue biopsy is accompanied by pathological and anatomical evidence, liquid biopsy obtains analytes from indirect body fluids such as the blood, urine, or saliva. Therefore, mechanistic studies confirming the tumor origin of these signals are the starting point for clinical application. Even if high sensitivity and specificity are reported, it cannot be assumed that the results directly reflect tumor status [15]. Rushing clinical application without mechanistic causality may lead to distorted treatment decisions and unnecessary consumption of medical resources.

cfDNA and ctDNA exemplify these challenges. Proposed release pathways include apoptosis, necrosis, and active secretion, but the dominant pathway in a given context depends on factors such as tumor stage, metastatic site, metabolic activity, and angiogenic status [16]. In anatomical barrier sites such as the brain, peritoneum, and bone metastases, ctDNA release into the bloodstream is restricted, and thus, ctDNA concentrations in blood may be low despite high disease activity [17]. This characteristic demonstrates that simple numerical interpretation can lead to erroneous conclusions.

The manner in which intra-tumoral heterogeneity is reflected also remains unclear. There is ongoing debate as to whether all subclones release ctDNA proportionally or whether clones with greater vascular access are overrepresented. If DNA from highly vascularized clones is preferentially reflected, the analysis may not represent the entire tumor but instead be biased toward specific clones. This issue can directly undermine the reliability of ctDNA-based predictive models.

Extracellular vesicles (EVs) face similar challenges. EVs can be secreted by various cell types and stably carry proteins, nucleic acids, and lipids, providing valuable information. However, markers that reliably distinguish tumor-derived EVs have yet to be established. Attempts have been made to use specific miRNAs or tetraspanin proteins as EV-based markers in prostate and pancreatic cancers, but discrimination from EVs originating from immune cells, platelets, hepatocytes, and other sources remains insufficient. Recent advances in EV research have identified large EVs known as blebbisomes, which have been found to contain various immunosuppressive proteins such as PD-L1, B7-H3, and HLA-E [18, 19]. Blebbisomes can reach sizes up to 20 μm and are suggested to function as central hubs in tumor-immune system interactions. This indicates that EV-based analysis may serve not only to provide tumor information but also as a means to explore key mediators of complex pathophysiology, such as immune evasion and resistance to immune checkpoint inhibitors (ICIs).

In conclusion, elucidating the mechanisms of analyte release and clearance is not merely a matter of technical performance improvement, but a fundamental task underpinning the interpretive reliability of liquid biopsy. Unless it is clearly established at the preclinical and basic research levels when and by what routes cfDNA, ctDNA, CTCs, and EVs are released into body fluids, and what factors govern their clearance or modification, clinical interpretability will remain limited. Interpretation requires not only describing the detection of analytes, but also scientifically explaining why, when, and how these substances are released into and cleared from body fluids. Therefore, research into these biological mechanisms should be regarded as the scientific evidence for all liquid biopsy interpretation and must be accumulated as a prerequisite for clinical translation.

8.7 Compliance with Regulatory Agency Guidelines

For liquid biopsy technologies to be adopted as practical tools in clinical settings, it is absolutely essential to meet the requirements of regulatory agencies, regardless of technical excellence. No matter how innovative an analytical platform may be, without robust, multilayered evidence for analytical validity, clinical validity, and clinical utility, it will face fundamental barriers to obtaining approval from regulatory bodies such as the FDA, EMA, or MFDS, or to being included in reimbursement systems.

As representative examples, Guardant360® CDx and FoundationOne® Liquid CDx received

FDA approval as companion diagnostics based on their ability to detect actionable mutations such as EGFR, BRAF, KRAS, and BRCA1/2. In this process, simply demonstrating high sensitivity and specificity was not sufficient. Strict analytical criteria had to be met. These included large-scale prospective and retrospective clinical trials involving thousands of patients, reproducibility testing across repeated measurements, evaluation of inter-sample variability, and inter-laboratory comparability. Such regulatory procedures are essential gateways for liquid biopsy technologies to be recognized as official medical practices that influence therapeutic decision-making, beyond their use as research tools.

Reimbursement is also a decisive factor in the dissemination and adoption of these technologies. The U.S. Centers for Medicare & Medicaid Services (CMS) issued a National Coverage Determination (NCD) for Guardant360 and FoundationOne Liquid CDx, establishing nationwide reimbursement criteria. Subsequently, private insurers also adopted coverage for these tests, significantly improving patient access to liquid biopsy. In contrast, other healthcare systems such as those in Korea and Europe require additional health economic evidence based on cost-effectiveness, long-term survival benefits, and patient-centered outcomes. Therefore, reducing the cost per test, generating real-world data (RWD) on actual patient survival improvement, and developing health economic models remain critical prerequisites for global adoption of liquid biopsy.

Furthermore, because liquid biopsy involves handling sensitive genomic information, ethical, legal, and social implications (ELSIs) constitute another important dimension. This includes data protection and de-identification, the scope and procedures for informed consent, addressing information asymmetry due to uncertainty in result interpretation, and ensuring equitable access to testing. For example, when variants such as BRCA1/2 or TP53—directly linked to familial or hereditary cancer syndromes—are detected, ethical guidelines are needed on how to communicate and manage this information with patients and their families.

Recently, concerns have been raised in the United States that subsequent clinical interventions based on liquid biopsy results, if implemented without sufficient validation, may lead to medical overaction. As a result, the establishment of trust-based governance systems and responsible implementation under regulatory guidance are being emphasized. Ultimately, for liquid biopsy to realize its true clinical value, scientific innovation must be accompanied by regulatory and ethical frameworks that ensure its safe and responsible integration into healthcare systems.

This work aims to provide a comprehensive foundation for understanding liquid biopsy, covering its conceptual and technological advances, characteristics of various analytes, clinical applications, pre-analytical and interpretive strategies, as well as its roles in companion diagnostics, MRD monitoring, and detection of resistance mechanisms. Despite the many challenges that remain, the potential of liquid biopsy is clear, and it is expected to evolve beyond precision medicine into new paradigms such as predictive medicine, patient-centered care, and real-time monitoring-based therapeutic decision-making. In particular, for treatments grounded in molecular evidence, such as immunotherapy or targeted therapy, liquid biopsy can serve as a dynamic and sensitive window reflecting the molecular and biological characteristics of disease, therapeutic response, and the emergence of resistance.

However, this ideal scenario cannot be achieved by technological excellence alone. As discussed in the main text, only when various considerations—such as analytical reliability, clinical applicability, cost-effectiveness, biological rationale, and regulatory and ethical compliance—are met, can liquid biopsy truly establish itself as a core tool of precision medicine, enabling genuinely personalized diagnosis and treatment. No longer merely a technical alternative, liquid biopsy acts as a catalyst driving a paradigm shift in cancer therapy, possessing the power to reshape the future of medicine around the patient. Rather than simply serving as a substitute or supplement to traditional diagnostic methods, liquid biopsy provides a precise window for interpreting the temporal and spatial complexity of tumor biology in a patient-specific manner.

References

1. Wan JCM, Massie C, Garcia-Corbacho J, Mouliere F, Brenton JD, Caldas C, et al. Liquid biopsies come of age: towards implementation of circulating tumour DNA. Nat Rev Cancer. 2017;17(4):223–38.
2. Cescon DW, Bratman SV, Chan SM, Siu LL. Circulating tumor DNA and liquid biopsy in oncology. Nat Cancer. 2020;1(3):276–90.
3. Merker JD, Oxnard GR, Compton C, Diehn M, Hurley P, Lazar AJ, et al. Circulating tumor DNA analysis in patients with cancer: American Society of Clinical Oncology and College of American Pathologists Joint Review. J Clin Oncol [Internet]. 2018 [cited 2025 Apr 29]. Available from: https://ascopubs.org/doi/10.1200/JCO.2017.76.8671.
4. Pantel K, Alix-Panabières C. Minimal residual disease as a target for liquid biopsy in patients with solid tumours. Nat Rev Clin Oncol. 2025;22(1):65–77.
5. Heitzer E, Haque IS, Roberts CES, Speicher MR. Current and future perspectives of liquid biopsies in genomics-driven oncology. Nat Rev Genet. 2019;20(2):71–88.
6. Alix-Panabières C, Pantel K. Liquid biopsy: from discovery to clinical application. Cancer Discov. 2021;11(4):858–73.
7. Lampignano R, Neumann MHD, Weber S, Kloten V, Herdean A, Voss T, et al. Multicenter evaluation of circulating cell-free DNA extraction and downstream analyses for the development of standardized (pre)analytical work flows. Clin Chem. 2020;66(1):149–60.
8. Schrag D, Beer TM, McDonnell CH, Nadauld L, Dilaveri CA, Reid R, et al. Blood-based tests for multicancer early detection (PATHFINDER): a prospective cohort study. Lancet. 2023;402(10409):1251–60.
9. Giridhar KV, Demeure MJ, Kim RH, Chen JA, Gadgeel S, Kurbegov D, et al. Abstract 4784: PATHFINDER 2: a prospective study to evaluate safety and performance of a multi-cancer early detection test in a population setting. Cancer Res. 2024;84(6_Supplement):4784.
10. Liu MC, Oxnard GR, Klein EA, Swanton C, Seiden MV, CCGA Consortium. Sensitive and specific multi-cancer detection and localization using methylation signatures in cell-free DNA. Ann Oncol. 2020;31(6):745–59.
11. Alix-Panabières C, Pantel K. Challenges in circulating tumour cell research. Nat Rev Cancer. 2014;14(9):623–31.
12. Lennon AM, Buchanan AH, Kinde I, Warren A, Honushefsky A, Cohain AT, et al. Feasibility of blood testing combined with PET-CT to screen for cancer and guide intervention. Science. 2020;369(6499):eabb9601.
13. Cohen JD, Li L, Wang Y, Thoburn C, Afsari B, Danilova L, et al. Detection and localization of surgically resectable cancers with a multi-analyte blood test. Science. 2018;359(6378):926–30.
14. Cristiano S, Leal A, Phallen J, Fiksel J, Adleff V, Bruhm DC, et al. Genome-wide cell-free DNA fragmentation in patients with cancer. Nature. 2019;570(7761):385–9.
15. Jahr S, Hentze H, Englisch S, Hardt D, Fackelmayer FO, Hesch RD, et al. DNA fragments in the blood plasma of cancer patients: quantitations and evidence for their origin from apoptotic and necrotic cells. Cancer Res. 2001;61(4):1659–65.
16. Thierry AR, El Messaoudi S, Gahan PB, Anker P, Stroun M. Origins, structures, and functions of circulating DNA in oncology. Cancer Metastasis Rev. 2016;35(3):347–76.
17. De Mattos-Arruda L, Mayor R, Ng CKY, Weigelt B, Martínez-Ricarte F, Torrejon D, et al. Cerebrospinal fluid-derived circulating tumour DNA better represents the genomic alterations of brain tumours than plasma. Nat Commun. 2015;6(1):8839.
18. Chen G, Huang AC, Zhang W, Zhang G, Wu M, Xu W, et al. Exosomal PD-L1 contributes to immunosuppression and is associated with anti-PD-1 response. Nature. 2018;560(7718):382–6.
19. Jeppesen DK, Sanchez ZC, Kelley NM, Hayes JB, Ambroise J, Koory EN, et al. Blebbisomes are large, organelle-rich extracellular vesicles with cell-like properties. Nat Cell Biol. 2025;27(3):438–48.

MIX
Papier aus verantwortungsvollen Quellen
Paper from responsible sources
FSC® C105338

If you have any concerns about our products,
you can contact us on
ProductSafety@springernature.com

In case Publisher is established outside the EU,
the EU authorized representative is:
Springer Nature Customer Service Center GmbH
Europaplatz 3, 69115 Heidelberg, Germany

Printed by Libri Plureos GmbH
in Hamburg, Germany